W9-BUO-813

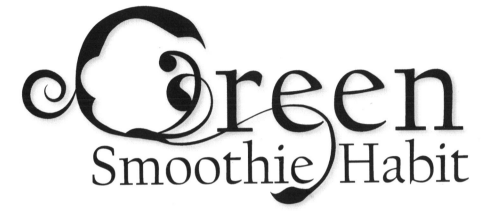

Green
Smoothie Habit

Drink Your Greens To Achieve Your Dreams

28 Day Success Guide

Jane Haddad

Green Smoothie Habit: Drink Your Greens To Achieve Your Dreams, 28 Day Success Guide

Copyright © 2013 by Jane Haddad

All rights reserved. No part of this book may be reproduced or transmitted in any form or by any means, electronic or mechanical, including photocopying, recording, printing, or by any information storage and retrieval system, without the permission in writing from the author.

ISBN 10: 0615842550
ISBN 13: 978-0615842554

Edited by Amber Haddad
Photography by Judith Phaneuf
Designed by Andrea Phaneuf

FIRST EDITION

Printed in the USA

Jane Haddad
P.O. Box 65304
Tucson, AZ 85728-5304
USA

www.GreenSmoothieHabit.com

To my husband Ron
and my children Amber and Cameron
You know why

To my sister Tammie
I miss you

TABLE OF CONTENTS

WELCOME LETTER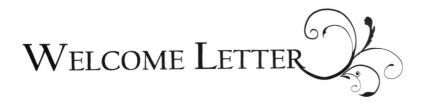

Your presence here defines you as a pioneer, taking your first steps in a brand new world to better health inside and out. Welcome to **Green Smoothie Habit**: Drink Your Greens To Achieve Your Dreams.

I wrote this book because there's more to greens than physical nutrition, as I reveal in Chapter 1 Discover The Code. I also introduce you to your lumen, explain what it is and how nourishing your lumen helps you achieve your dreams.

I designed this book to be interactive. I want you to write in it, bookmark it and keep it in the kitchen next to your blender. Each section has a purpose and is carefully planned to keep you engaged and increase your chances of earning your Certificate Of Achievement.

I've written you notes along the way that give you insight into my green smoothie experience and are meant, along with the Thought Of The Day, to educate and inspire. The Action Steps are thoughtful and doable, build upon each other and help you create your green smoothie habit.

I include information and a photograph about each green so that you can get to know them, understand why they are beneficial and be able to identify them when shopping. Practical tips, green smoothie menus, shopping lists and built-in inspiration support your efforts. Also, my online community, GreenSmoothieHabit.com/myHabit, awaits you.

Lettuce drink our greens to achieve our dreams,

Jane

Disclaimer

Do Not Construe as Medical Advice or Treatment

All content herein is the sole opinion of the author and in no way is intended to be or should be construed as medical advice or treatment. The reader of this information is solely responsible for his or her actions and the consequences thereof. If you want, need or seek medical advice or treatment, see a doctor.

The techniques and advice described in this book represent the opinions of the author based on her experience. The author expressly disclaims any responsibility for any liability, loss or risk, personal or otherwise, which is incurred as a result of using any of the techniques, tools, recipes or recommendations suggested herein. If in any doubt, or if requiring medical advice, please contact the appropriate health professional.

Acknowledgements

Andrea Phaneuf, Book and Web Designer, Food Stylist, whose spirit and artistry inspired me to make the content worthy of her design. Without her assistance and guidance this book would not have been possible.

Judith Phaneuf, Photographer, whose author photographs and images of the greens bring with them her personal code of vision, passion and ethics.

Amber Haddad, Melissa Lal, Kris Marsh, Judith Phaneuf, and Ariel Policano ND, whose willingness to read my drafts and give candid commentary helped me bring you a better book.

And to the thousands of men and women who visit GreenSmoothieHabit. com and watch my videos, make the recipes, share their thoughts and reviews and come back for more with their support and love. Thank you from the bottom of my blender.

ABOUT THE AUTHOR

Jane Haddad is the founder of GreenSmoothieHabit.com where she provides videos, recipes, support, motivation, inspiration and instruction for all who seek to drink their greens to achieve their dreams.

Jane has been creating, consuming, writing about, teaching and enjoying the benefits of green smoothies since 2006. Jane is not a doctor or nutritionist and holds no degrees. She resides in Arizona with her husband, drinks green smoothies and has fun with family and friends.

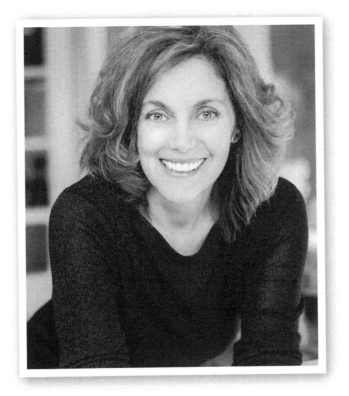

"My blender is my #1 wellbeing tool. When I'm drinking my greens, I feel 18 again."

-Jane

Introduction

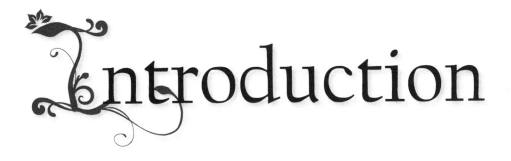

INTRODUCTION

"Start somewhere, do something."
—Jane

My earliest memory of thinking about food and losing weight was at 11 years old. Why was I wrapped up in what I ate and how I looked at the age of 11?

All through my teen years, my twenties and thirties, my forties and now, it's been about food. Food as comfort, food as killer, food as cure.

I've been an emotional binge eater, an ice cream eater, a starvation diet non-eater. I have formally fasted and received my certificate from the Ancient Accepted Order of Hygienic Fasters in 1978. Yes, I existed on pure water alone for 25 days and was recognized for "unusual merit and self-discipline."

I was liberated from my food issues by drinking my greens. Fresh, leafy greens. I didn't know I would receive this important benefit from the greens. That I could drink my greens and forget about the rest of it, but that's what has happened. It's called food freedom.

Fresh greens let me out of my food jail. Drinking my greens has solved my food issues like nothing else. I actually go for days without thinking about food in any other way than, wow, I enjoy my fresh foods. I feel good, my energy is liberated, I am positive and cheerful.

I developed **Green Smoothie Habit** from all of my life experience, not just food. All of us are bodies of work and knowledge. We are tested and overcome difficulties, which results in hard won experience. What to do with that experience? In this case, I developed GreenSmoothieHabit.com so I could share what I have learned and help others to drink their greens to achieve their dreams. It is so satisfying to make this kind of progress.

I see no reason why you can't make progress, too.

MY STORY

The reason I began drinking my greens was because my sister Tammie, who I've dedicated this book to, died from invasive breast cancer. I was so traumatized by her death and her 16 month journey leading up to it, that all I could think about was cancer. I checked my body for it, thought every ache and pain was it, and searched for ways to prevent it.

During my search, I came across a vital piece of the cancer prevention puzzle: Victoria Boutenko's *Green For Life*, which contained, for me, a life changing excerpt on page 80:

 OWEVER, I think the main reason for illness was stated very clearly in 1931! Over 75 years ago Otto Warburg was awarded the Nobel prize for his discovery that cancer is caused by weakened cell respiration due to lack of oxygen at the cellular level.

Three words stayed with me from Boutenko's *Green For Life*:

greens,

chlorophyll,

oxygen.

My primary goal became to create the chlorophyll and oxygen rich environment that keeps cancer from thriving.

Greens help me do that.

And although there are no guarantees of anything for any of us, I began drinking my greens as a cancer prevention measure and as a way to heal my broken heart. Little did I know what would unfold. Little did I know greens contain the code and lumen to connect the dots between plant and human.

As for the various eating and food programs I put myself on during my adult life, they all failed because they didn't include fresh, leafy greens. Unadulterated, undressed, unoiled, unsauced, uncooked, unsalted, undisguised greens.

As for cancer, we may have it dormant in our bodies. The key is to nurture its sleep, not its awakening.

WHAT ARE YOU?

We'll get into who you are in Chapter 3 Through The Portal, as the answer to that question is within you and nowhere else. But the answer to the question "What are you?" will clarify why drinking your greens can help you.

The answer will keep you motivated.

The answer is the engine of wellbeing.

The answer is one word.

water

You are *water*

- Your blood is 83% *water*.

- Your muscles are 75% *water*.

- Your brain is 74% *water*.

- Your bones are 22% *water*.

Simple. You are water.

So ingest high water content foods. The easiest way to do this is through green smoothies. They contain an abundance of high water content fresh fruits and the magic of fresh, leafy greens.

WHY ARE GREENS MAGICAL?

Greens are magical because they contain the code, which is more than physical nutrition, as revealed in Chapter 1 Discover The Code.

Greens deliver naturally purified water, as detailed in the Nutritional Data section in the Appendix.

Greens contain vital components our bodies yearn for and are delighted with, including vitamins, minerals and essential amino acids, featured in Chapter 2 Meet the Greens. How do I know my body is delighted when I drink greens? I experience it. I have lived life Before Greens and After Greens.

WHY BLEND?

The primary purpose of blending is because high speed blenders break down the cellular walls of greens and unleash the sun kissed, soil nourished, mineral dense food so that it passes effortlessly through our digestive membranes and into our blood stream.

The secondary purpose of blending is so that we can easily and tastily consume fresh, leafy greens without oils and salt, enjoying them in their alkaline state. This helps diminish cell degeneration, provide essential water content, maintain correct blood pH and reduce inflammation.

They create an "all is well with the world" disposition in me, and if that were the only thing greens did, I'd be satisfied.

COLON

Wellbeing begins in the bowel and generally speaking, bowel health means daily elimination. Are you regular? If not enough is coming out, or not often enough, or too often, or too much like slurry, or too much like cardboard, then your colon is warning you of trouble ahead.

We are starting from the inside out. Inner cleanliness and calm.

Think of it as cleaning out your closets of clutter and decades old clothes that no longer work. It's a new beginning with a designed–just–for–you couture wardrobe. We know when our closets or colons are clogged. We know what results from constipated closets and colons.

Lettuce drink our greens and feel the gentle spa rinse as the chlorophyll in the greens purifies our inner terrain, enriches and nourishes our red blood cells, strengthens our immune system and carries iron and oxygen to our cells.

FIBER

Can we speak of inner cleanliness and calm without speaking of fiber? No.

We all know that fiber promotes regularity. But did you also know that fiber promotes healthy intestinal bacteria, binds carcinogens and curbs overeating? Green smoothies are rich in chlorophyll, oxygen, water and fiber; the engine of wellbeing.

The friendly fiber in greens provides bulk and sweeps detritus onward to the bowel and out of the body, providing us with cleanliness and good cheer. The results of plant fiber goodness must be experienced to be appreciated and green smoothies are an easy and simple way to respect our alimentary canal while satisfying our nutritional needs and pleasing our taste buds.

You have been introduced to the
green smoothie habit.

Let's discover the code...

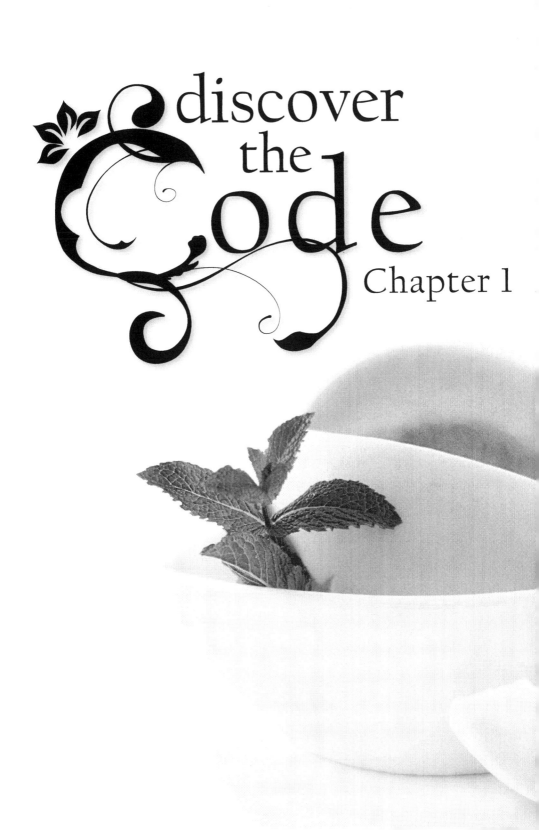

discover the Code

Chapter 1

1 | Discover the Code
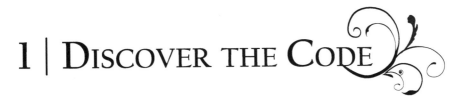

"Overcome adversity by nourishing your inner strength and finding out what is true."

–Jane

My True Hunger

Drinking my greens has become a habit in my life. Greens not only nourish my body, they nourish my soul and feed my true hunger – the hunger for inspiration, consolation and satisfaction. The purpose of my four week guide is to lay the foundation so that you, too, can make drinking your greens a habit in your life.

Fresh, leafy greens help liberate my energy, dissolve my belly fat, ward off cravings, stabilize my emotions, pace my progress and help me to see projects through, one step at a time, to satisfying completion.

Can you achieve all this in 28 days? No. At the time of this writing, I have been drinking my greens for 7 years. But what you can achieve in 28 days is to establish the foundation and create the habit of drinking your greens.

When your 28 days are over, I hope you will continue to drink your greens and be served by the code.

Follow me...

ABOUT THE CODE

There is an open space called **lumen**, the Latin word for light, that exists in our blood vessels and intestines. When a hollow organ is sliced crosswise, you can see light through the space that has been opened. This light is your lumen and it surrounds and contains your blood.

Lumen also exists in plants and is the light filled cavity surrounded by the plant's cell wall.

We both contain lumen and that's the connection. That's where plant light and human light merge, in our lumen. I have discovered that by drinking my greens I can harvest the plant's light.

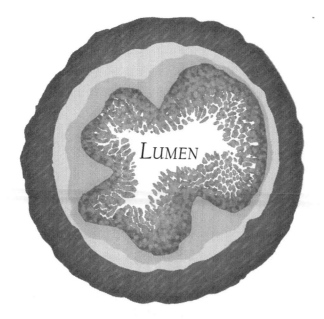

HIGHER REASON

This discovery has made it possible for me to have a higher reason for drinking my greens, and the long term drinking of greens has benefited my body and mind.

One of the most important benefits I have experienced is the inner strength to replace fear with action, grief with purpose and midlife invisibility with a vibrant new view. Those are big. Did you notice none of them are about food? Drinking my greens has opened up a sunlit, luminescent space within me. It's irresistible and it beckons.

It's exhilarating to learn about myself in this way. I see no reason why it can't happen for you. Drinking your greens will inform you and eventually enable you to replace fear with action. No matter how little or seemingly inconsequential, each positive action you take in the direction you dream of heading will nourish you in a way no food or drink ever could. That includes greens, which are your food foundation for positive action, which keeps you drinking your greens. It's an exciting circle.

NOURISH YOUR LUMEN

Not only is lumen the Latin word for light, but it is also the word for opening. It is a physical reality, the lumen that resides in us and plants. It is not some far off science fiction.

When we drink our greens we are drinking sunlight, which is absorbed by our bloodstream, nourishing our lumen and intensifying the light radiating outward through the surface of our body. This light is expressed by our mindset and measured by our actions.

I have also found that drinking my greens nourishes my courage. I have no scientific proof. I don't need any. I know from living it. From putting greens in my blender in umpteen combinations on a consistent basis since 2006. I know from being imperfect, fully flawed and staying hungry. I want. I want. I want. How hungry are you? You'd better be starving or you will never replace fear with positive action.

It won't happen by reading my words. You must buy fresh greens. You must blend them. You must sip and savor them. On the next page, I illustrate how I envision the code: the more greens you consume, the sunnier your lumen forecast.

THE CODE

Daily Greens Consumed		Lumen Forecast	
	Prepare for Planetary Travel		☐
	Sunny Inside and Out		☐
	Partially Sunny		☐
	Cloudy		☐
	Darkness		☐

~400g | ~200g | ~100g | ~50g

A CTION STEP:

Check the forecast box that best describes your lumen now.

YOUR GREEN SMOOTHIE HABIT

You may experience some or all of the following during your 28 days:

- Lose an inch or two of your belly fat
- Lose four to eight pounds
- See your skin begin to glow
- Feel radiantly beautiful
- Experience your bowels regulate
- Provide sagging skin the inner hydration it needs to plump
- Wake up in the morning with decreased or no mucous
- Experience more energy, which, long dormant, begins to stir
- Experience more positive moods
- Experience more generous attitudes
- Enjoy fresher breath and reduced body odor
- Learn patience when Mother Nature does things her way and not your way

Results are not average or limited to the above list, as I don't know what condition you are in, where you are starting from or how far you want to go. Don't expect miracles, but do expect progress.

A common question: What can I do to stay on plan so I don't stray?

I used to be concerned about that, too, but I no longer think straying is bad. I think it's necessary and I think it delivers to us valuable emotional information and in many cases valuable nutrients.

What is straying? It is different for each of us. It depends on how we manage our expectations and on why we want to drink our greens. Our purpose here is to develop the habit of drinking fresh, leafy greens, not to attain the unattainable or to punish ourselves for straying.

I'm serious when I say drink your greens and forget about the rest of it. This can be difficult for those of us who have spent our lives dogmatic about food plans and diets, afraid to fail and we always do. Please allow yourself failure. The more failure, the more experience. The more experience, the more knowing. The more knowing, the more success.

For me, **Green Smoothie Habit** is about building a nutritional foundation from which I can overcome my fears and achieve my dreams. It is so nourishing to overcome a fear and replace it with a positive action. Drinking my greens helps me accomplish that and I wrote **Green Smoothie Habit** to help you accomplish it, too.

Stray? I say stray far and wide, for your straying is life itself trying to unleash you and force you to see yourself in a new way – by the light of your sunlit lumen.

You have discovered the code.

Let's meet the greens...

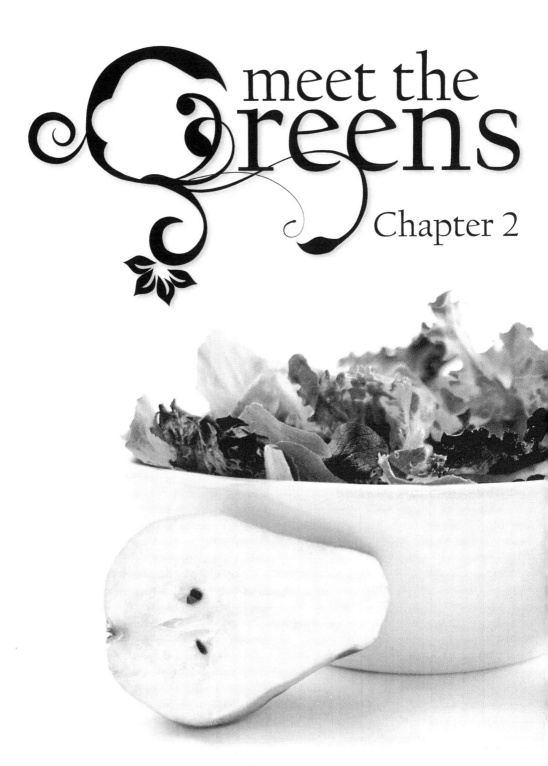

meet the Greens

Chapter 2

2 | MEET THE GREENS

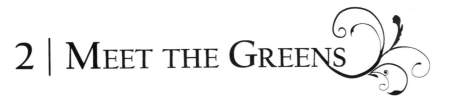

"Drink your greens to achieve your dreams."

—Jane

When I drink my greens, I feel good.

I feel good while I'm shopping for greens, because the produce area is the most beautiful and vibrant part of the grocery store and I feel alive when I'm in it.

I feel good while I'm blending the fresh greens and fruit, because of the colors and aroma released by the blender.

I feel good while I'm sipping and savoring my green smoothie, all lit up inside.

Greens treat me well and I feel good eating and drinking them. Positivity and cheer fill me. Life isn't perfect and every minute isn't roses, but many are. Enough for me to keep drinking my greens.

Allow me to introduce you to the components of your life building, energy releasing, beauty enhancing green goodness team...

COMPONENTS OF THE GREENS

Essential Amino Acids

Fresh, leafy greens are abundant in virgin amino acids waiting to be consumed by you so they can construct the perfect protein for you. Who doesn't want their very own custom protein to help them have the best health and wellbeing, beauty, form and function?

Consuming a wide variety of fresh, leafy greens provides the 9 essential amino acids we cannot produce and must consume. They are essential for human life and come with exotic names like Histidine, Phenylalanine and Valine.

Consider them your in-house design team, working exclusively for you around the clock to make you the strongest, most powerful, most beautiful, perfect protein creature on God's green earth. All they ask is that you give them something to work with:

 HISTIDINE: For your sexual arousal and pleasure, healthy tissues throughout the body, and especially the myelin sheaths that provide a protective layer around nerve cells.

 ISOLEUCINE: Excels at the production and maintenance of body proteins, regulates metabolism, the thymus gland in the neck, the spleen, pituitary glands and hemoglobin production.

LEUCINE: Increases production of growth hormones and helps break down visceral fat, which is the belly fat that surrounds the internal organs and is the least responsive to diet and exercise.

*L*YSINE: Necessary for proper collagen formation and the abundant protein that makes up our bones, cartilage, ligaments and tendons.

*M*ETHIONINE: Excellent source of sulfur used to promote hair, skin and nail growth. Sulfur also helps reduce liver fat and cholesterol, eliminates heavy metals and toxins and protects the kidneys.

*P*HENYLALANINE: For the normal functioning of our central nervous system and the making of our neurotransmitters, which send information to and from our brain's nerve cells.

*T*HREONINE: Promotes proper protein balance in the body and supports cardiovascular, liver, central nervous and immune system function. Helps maintain strong, elastic tissues and muscles, including the heart.

*T*RYPTOPHAN: Plays an important role in the production of nervous system messengers, especially those related to relaxation, restfulness and sleep.

*V*ALINE: Promotes tissue growth and repair, regulates blood sugar, provides the body with energy, helps to stimulate the central nervous system and is needed for proper mental functioning.

Minerals

Minerals help your body grow and stay strong and healthy. As with the 9 essential amino acids, our bodies can't produce minerals. We have to consume them.

Fresh, leafy greens are stunners in their mineral content and delivery. Do you want to be stunning? Get your greens.

If you rotate your greens as advised and get a wide variety on a consistent basis, you will be getting some or all of the following potent minerals, vital to your team:

CALCIUM
The chief constituent for strong bones, teeth and the prevention of osteoporosis.

COPPER
Is crucial for metabolic health, brain stimulation and normal growth.

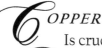
IRON
Boosts the body's energy, improves immunity and encourages sound sleep.

MAGNESIUM
Stabilizes transmission of nerve impulses, body temperature regulation and energy production.

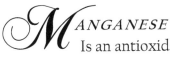ANGANESE
Is an antioxidant, free radical fighting micronutrient important for food digestion and bone structure.

HOSPHORUS
Works with Calcium to build strong bones and teeth and maintain tissue health.

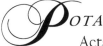OTASSIUM
Acts as an electrolyte keeping the heart, brain, kidney and muscle tissues healthy.

ELENIUM
Is a trace mineral found in healthy soil, naturally appears in water and plays a key role in metabolism and antioxidant enzymes.

ODIUM
Helps maintain the balance of positive and negative ions in body fluids and tissues.

INC
Found in every tissue of the body, it is a powerful antioxidant and helps maintain hormone levels.

Vitamins

Vitamins help us prevent deficiencies and reduce the risk of developing various diseases and disorders. They are essential for normal metabolism and are found in whole foods and fresh, leafy greens.

One of the best aspects of getting a wide variety of greens is the pristine, full spectrum vitamins they deliver on a silver platter to you, for you. Graciously accept their gifts:

 RETINOL
Is essential for our white blood cells which fight infection in our body.

 1 THIAMIN
Keeps mucous membranes healthy and is responsible for converting sugar into energy.

 2 RIBOFLAVIN
Helps produce red blood cells, protects the nervous system and breaks down fats, proteins and carbohydrates for energy.

 3 NIACIN
Helps the body convert food into fuel and makes sex and stress related hormones in the adrenal glands.

PANTOTHENIC ACID
Produces neurotransmitters in the brain,
fabricates steroids and extracts fats,
proteins and vital nutrients.

 PYRIDOXINE
Is involved in more bodily functions than
any other single nutrient and functions as a
coenzyme in more than 100 bodily processes.

 FOLATE
Prevents birth defects in the fetus,
strengthens the nervous system and
produces healthy red blood cells.

 ASCORBIC ACID
Protects the body from infection and
strengthens the immune system.

 TOCOPHEROL
Helps prevent inflammation, mental
deterioration and scarring of skin.

 PHYTONADIONE
Helps maintain a healthy blood clotting
system and keeps blood vessels from
calcifying.

Oxygen

The Beating Heart of Your Greens Team

Greens enrich our blood, which carries life giving oxygen to our cells. No longer will your cells be gasping for air. With each sip of a green smoothie, cells alkalinize, lymph fluid aerates and circulates and hemoglobin counts are built.

I can say from experience that I feel light radiating inside my abdomen when I am drinking my greens. I believe it comes not only from my lumen being nourished but by my cells achieving full hydration and oxygen, getting great gulps of pure water and air thanks to the greens.

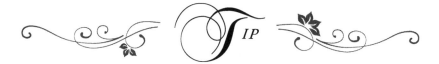

TIP

For your convenience, the Nutritional Data section in the Appendix lists the nutrient values for the fresh greens and herbs used in **Green Smoothie Habit**. Listed for each green are:

* Water
* Minerals
* Calories
* Vitamins
* Protein
* Essential Amino Acids

HEALTH BENEFITS YOU MAY ENJOY

PURIFYING SKIN with PURIFIED WATER

Greens have high water content and this naturally purified water...

- nourishes and plumps skin
- helps prevent dehydration
- helps prevent loss of elasticity
- helps eliminate toxins eaten and absorbed
- helps you feel happy, hydrated and youthful
- moisturizes at the cellular level, hair, eyes and skin glow

CLEANSING with CHLOROPHYLL

Greens are bursting with chlorophyll, the green pigment found in plants that allows...

- plants to derive energy from light, which transfers to us
- essential oxygen to be carried to our cells
- body odors to be reduced
- inflammation to be calmed
- harmful bacteria to be eliminated
- lumen to be nourished, strengthening our light

POSITIVITY and CHEER

Greens enable mindfulness and conscious health choices...

- encouraging wellbeing, resulting in being well
- cleansing not clogging, healing not harming
- building muscle, mental might and emotional fortitude
- freeing and fortifying your whole being
- regulating the bowels
- freeing up time and unleashing dreams

GREEN GOODNESS GOODIES

Greens have many positive aspects and are...

- rich in essential amino acids, vitamins, minerals and fiber
- low glycemic and help balance energy levels
- naturally probiotic, promoting good intestinal flora
- helpful in regulating blood pressure, fluid levels and muscle control
- helpful in keeping common colds and daily irritations away
- rich in B–carotene and Vitamin C, supporting your immune, cardiovascular and nervous systems

There's a lot of goodness in greens.

Now let's take a peek through the portal...

Chapter 3
Through
the portal

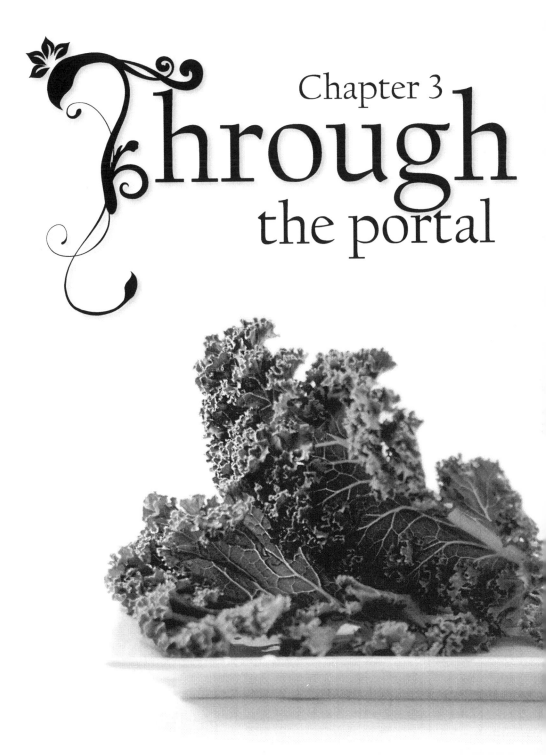

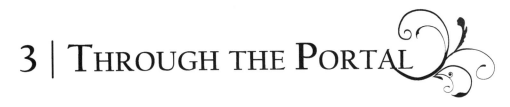

3 | THROUGH THE PORTAL

"Drinking your greens builds the inner strength that gives beauty its depth."

-Jane

There's a portal in fresh greens. I know because I've found it. Drinking your greens will help you through the portal to the other side where your dreams, motivation and inspiration dwell.

I've actually had a dream come true. The dream of creating my website where you can "drink your greens to achieve your dreams" has come true. It's not perfect, but it's here, thriving, and I am thrilled.

What is your dream? The one dream that must be achieved? The one that is you manifested in that crazy idea that yearns to be expressed? I ask you these questions because this book is as much about achieving your dreams as it is about building your green smoothie habit. They complement each other. If they didn't, I wouldn't be writing to you now, I wouldn't have made the connection, sipped the greens and achieved a dream.

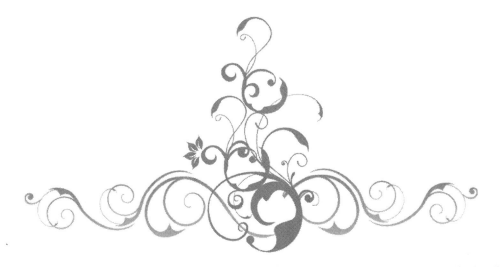

THE AMAZING THING

It's not only about the greens. It's about much more than food. It's about the code, lumen and the portal. I have walked through the portal that drinking sunshine creates, and on the other side I found the inner strength, the discipline and the joy that enables me to replace fear with action and put one foot in front of the other in the direction I dream of heading. I see no reason why that can't happen for you.

That's the amazing thing about drinking your greens. Yes, there are health benefits that I enjoy, the energy and the mental clarity foremost. But there are also the unseen benefits of being able to accomplish the work necessary to make a dream a reality. Drinking my greens not only nourishes my body, it nourishes my courage and inner strength.

Dreams

I'm not saying all dreams will come true for all people. That isn't the way it works. You have to be willing to work when you don't feel like it, stay enthused when you are not enthusiastic and work when others play. Achieving a dream happens when you take action to accomplish a chore, then rest and move on to the next task. Eventually you complete them all and are able to look at a whole, however imperfect. You continue working on it, improving and refining as you go, but not waiting to be perfect before you begin.

I have had many dreams. I used to begin with excitement, get a third or halfway through and then hit the middle, that long parched desert where it becomes really difficult to keep going. Usually at this point I would quit, never knowing what it was like to finish.

All that began to change slowly, so slowly, when I began to drink my greens. Will you quit the dream you are presently upon? Or will you continue to put one foot in front of the other in the direction you dream of heading?

Finishing

When one is in the clutch of reaching a goal, it is the finishing that is the hardest. I never really understood that during the many dreams I started but found myself unable to finish. All that quitting weakens a person and undermines one's confidence more than anything, because it is not done to us by others, we do it to ourselves.

When I allowed myself to begin imperfectly, remain imperfect, accept my imperfections, do what I could when I could, including the food part of my life, that is when my life began to relax and hum along. Imperfection is such a freedom.

I've been drinking my greens for seven years now and continue on imperfectly, letting my fears get puréed along with my greens in my blender.

The Code

Could I have accomplished food freedom and dream achievement without drinking my greens? No. I know that because for 40 years I tried all the plans and my behavior and health didn't change.

I now know what happened. I was drying up inside from inferior food choices and a weak will. When I added in the greens, my heart and mind slowly began to rehydrate and plump up with possibility. My skin became soft and smooth, my body leapt out of bed in the morning and began serving my dreams instead of my nightmares. My choice to drink my greens instigated a physiological change in me that affected my entire being.

The changes seemed chaotic and random, but as I look back I see the order in them. Suffice it to say that I am glad I allowed the greens to nourish me and I am grateful I was ready to accept the changes they instigated.

Change never looks and feels the way you think, and if you don't have the courage, it will go away. Nothing is more sad than being on the brink of self improvement but being too scared to let it happen. There's no telling when change will come back and try again, or if it ever will. My greens drinking helped to create the necessary courage to allow positive changes to happen.

WHAT IS YOUR DREAM?

Choose one dream and stick to it. Just one, even if it's no more than cleaning out a cluttered closet, losing that belly fat, writing a daily page of your great American novel or going parasailing and floating in the open sky of opportunity. Accomplish it.

Can I guarantee that your dreams will come true if you drink your greens? No, I can't. I can't even guarantee my own. What I do know is that drinking my greens has helped me make one dream come true. And if one dream can come true, so can two.

I don't know what you are seeking, but I do know that I can help you establish the habit of drinking your greens and if you already do, help you improve.

What do you want to find on the other side of the green smoothie portal?

So come on, be a pioneer.

*Take advantage of the support and motivation built in to **Green Smoothie Habit.***

While nothing's perfect, some things are a lot of fun!

do the plan
Chapter 4

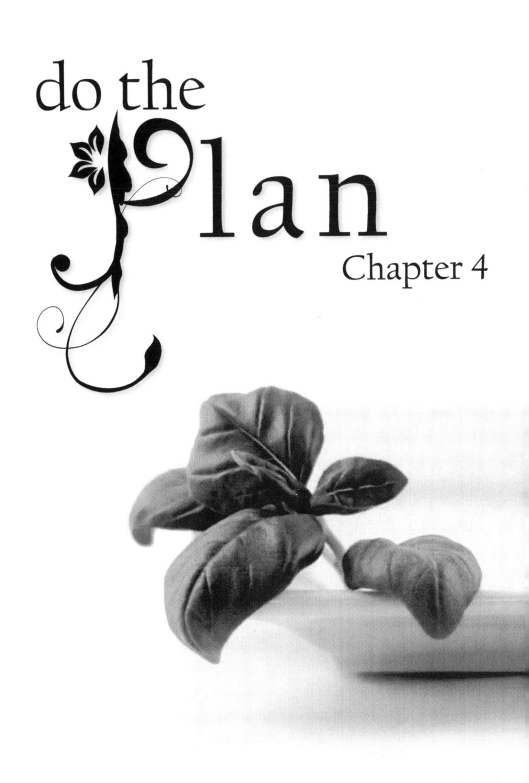

4 | DO THE PLAN

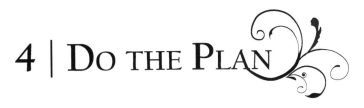

"Blend. Sip. Beautify."

-Jane

You have already started your **Green Smoothie Habit** by learning and getting your mind and body ready for the next 28 days. But here is where you really begin.

Offering

> "I enjoy being patient."

Say this aloud or to yourself whenever you feel the wellspring of impatience, anxiety or fear arising within you. They travel together like a pack of wolves, the three dream killers. Witness their instant dissolution as you state,

> "I enjoy being patient."

It works wonders and triggers a physical sigh of relief that will instantly relax you. I use this positive thought for all aspects of my life, not just food. These four powerful words have helped me replace my fear driven mindset with my take action mindset. I offer them to you.

Don't Panic

I am not asking you to stop eating anything in particular or to give up your favorite foods. I am not asking you to change. You won't have to do the work of change, as the greens do that.

I am asking you to take action. Chew a leaf of lettuce. Gnaw a cucumber. Make a lumpy green smoothie in an underpowered blender. Begin being well now.

We are all on our own journey in our own time. I know from experience that nothing happens a moment sooner, or a moment later, than it is supposed to. What a relief.

Tools & Tips

We all know the difference between simple and easy. The beautiful thing about drinking your greens is that it's simple and easy. How often in our lives does that happen?

Green smoothies are a fast, efficient, nutrient dense food and drink, meant to be sipped and savored, not gulped and gobbled. This way you can enjoy the unique mouth feel of green smoothies and also more tenderly introduce them into your system without surprises.

The greens I feature in my recipes are common, readily available greens. You don't have to shop in specialty markets or special order expensive, fancy items. Organic is best, but don't let it stop you from getting started.

Shopping

Don't overbuy. I learned this the hard way. There's nothing worse than stocking up only to watch your precious greens wilt, die and turn to slime. Extra greens that don't go into your smoothies can be used in salads, soups, sautés and steamed and baked dishes.

I realize everyone's situation is different: access to stores, time and energy, money and climate, but the rule holds. Buy what you know you can use, savor every sip, run out while you're still wanting more and look forward to buying and consuming more greens.

Rotate Your Greens

Today kale, tomorrow chard, etc. This is the most important tip I can give you. Greens contain alkaloids (poisonous substances produced by plants) and the human body has no trouble eliminating small amounts of them, but you don't want to build up a large store of any one of them. By rotating your greens, this won't happen.

In my four week guide, I have incorporated 20 common greens in 28 days, giving you a wide variety and showing you how to rotate your greens. If you don't want to use my recipes you don't have to, just use as wide a variety of greens as possible. Think 7 different greens in 7 days and that will help you rotate your greens in line with what is available in your area at any time.

Most markets carry over a dozen varieties, and greens are easy to find once you start looking. Try new ones.

You don't have to rotate fruit, as fruit doesn't contain alkaloids (except for tomatoes, which are a part of the nightshade family and do produce alkaloids). If you want to use mango, apples, melon or any fruit over and over, you can do that. It is your greens you must rotate, not your fruit.

Freshness and Storage

How do you know if greens are fresh? While in the store, hold them up by the rubber band or wire bundled stems, out in front of you like you're presenting someone with a bouquet of flowers. Do the leaves remain upright on their own or do they fall over like they are tired? If they're floppy, move on, even if you have to change your planned green for the day. Buy fresh and when you get them home, your greens drinking life will last longer, go smoother and taste better.

For the most part, I keep fresh greens in the vegetable bin or any of the temperature controlled or separate drawers in the refrigerator. I don't use frozen greens in my smoothies, but some people do and it is better to get frozen greens than no greens at all.

I do not prep my greens in the traditional sense of cleaning, trimming and storing in individual baggies so that they'll be ready. This step becomes unnecessary when you don't overbuy in the first place. Also, I find prepping fresh greens shortens their life and they wilt sooner. I wash what I need when I need it and it goes right in the blender. Easier, more efficient, simpler.

Clean Your Greens

Wash your greens and fruit before consuming them. Wash everything in a sink full of water and ½ cup of white distilled vinegar, swishing it around and getting rid of the anonymous hands, soil, bacteria and other unfriendly microorganisms that may be inhabiting it. Rinse well.

Clean produce is a joy to consume. Please don't think that because it's organic, it doesn't need washing. One just doesn't know what it has come into contact with before you get it home.

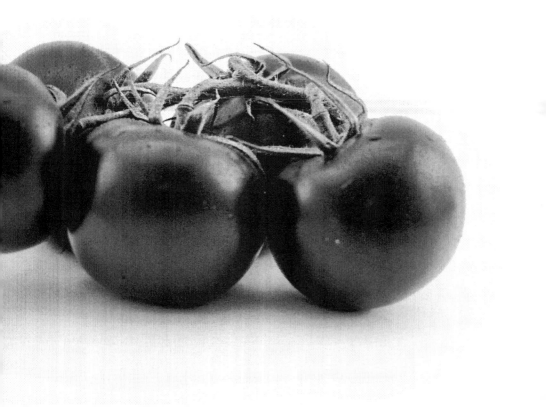

HOW TO BLEND GREEN SMOOTHIES

BLENDING DIRECTIONS

- Load ingredients into your blender as follows: liquids, fruit, then greens, then ice.
- Blend 45 seconds in a high speed blender. You're done.

FRUIT AND GREENS RATIO

- Don't want to follow recipes and measurements? Let ⅔ fruit, ⅓ greens be your guide.
- Substitute fruit and greens as you like.
- Mix, match and create your own signature green smoothies.
- Start with one leaf if that's all the green your taste buds can tolerate and build up from there.

BLEND TO YOUR TASTES

- Too green? Add fruit.
- Too sweet? Add greens.
- Add ice! Or water! Or not!

Recipes and Proportions

You don't have to use my green smoothie recipes. You can create your own blends if you like. Enjoy the art of green smoothie making.

Quantities of recipes vary from 2 cups to 7 cups. If need be, play with proportions to suit your situation. Share with family or reduce or alter quantities of fruit, greens and liquids. Or you can proportionally reduce quantities of greens and fruit by using the basic ⅔ fruit, ⅓ greens ratio. Whatever you do, get your greens.

Blenders

Green smoothies are best made in a high speed blender like a Vitamix®, but not required. If you don't have a high speed blender, work with what you have. You may have to cut the recipe in half or thirds or add more liquid or leave out the ice to get it to blend, and it may not be as smooth as you like, but that's okay. Do something, start somewhere.

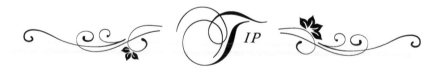

Apple seeds and seeded grapes, etc., are fine to use in a high speed blender, otherwise remove seeds and pits from fruit. For your convenience, see the Appendix, page 252 for a compilation of green smoothie making tips.

THE PREPARATION

Choose your start day 2–3 days out. This gives you time to peruse the weekly green smoothie recipes and do your shopping for week one. Get the simple ingredients in one shopping trip or spread it out between 2 or 3 trips to the market throughout the week, depending on what works for you. You will find a new menu and shopping list for each week.

THE SCHEDULE

Mornings

- Start each day by reviewing the Note from Jane, Thought of the Day, Recipe and Action Steps.

- Make your green smoothie.

- Sip and savor your green smoothie before ingesting other foods; this is preferable but not mandatory.

Evenings

- Complete your Action Steps. You will gain valuable insights as the days and weeks of drinking your greens add up.

- You can also make smoothies the night before and refrigerate, except for those using banana, consume those fresh.

THE PROMISE

Just promise me one thing. That you'll drink your greens. If you do none of the action steps, if you eschew the accountability, then just drink your greens. That's the easy and delicious part!

Here we go...

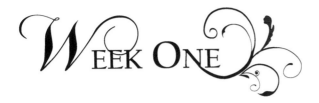

Week One

"You can do it."

–Jane

would have loved to have had all this mapped out for me when I was getting started, so I have mapped it out for you.

No matter where you are in your belly busting, energy releasing, courage seeking existence, **Green Smoothie Habit**: Drink Your Greens To Achieve Your Dreams can support and help you.

One day at a time, for 28 days, you will build the good and positive habit of drinking your greens. Be gentle with yourself as you proceed. We are human beings, not machines. During the next four weeks this book will help you find out how the code works for you and will guide you day by day and week by week, so that you don't get overwhelmed.

Change takes time. Not everything you want will happen in these 28 days. Simply enjoy the greens. The rest will happen for you in its own way and time. You're stronger than you think and you can do it.

MENU & SHOPPING LIST

DAY 1: **Who Knew? Green Smoothie**

DAY 2: **Feel Better Green Smoothie**

DAY 3: **Beautiful Skin Green Smoothie**

DAY 4: **Thirst Quencher Green Smoothie**

DAY 5: **Carrot Top Green Smoothie**

DAY 6: **Anti-Oxidant Green Smoothie**

DAY 7: **Cherry Chard Green Smoothie**

GREENS & VEGGIES

Iceburg Lettuce, ½ head (D1)

Lacinato/Dinosaur Kale, 2 – 3 leaves (D2)

Parsley, ¾ bunch *any variety* (D3)

Mint, 2 handfuls *fresh* (D3 & 5)

Romaine Lettuce, 4 – 6 leaves (D4)

Carrot Top/Greens, handful (D5)

Collard Greens, 2 – 3 leaves (D6)

Chard, 2 – 3 leaves (D7)

PANTRY

Sea Salt, ¼ t (D1)

Cinnamon, ½ t (D2)

FRUIT

Tomato, 1 (D1)

Cucumbers, 2 (D1 & 3)

Apple Juice, 4 c *fresh* (D2)

Lemon Juice, 2 T *fresh* (D2)

Grapefruit, 1 (D3)

Orange Juice, ½ c *fresh* (D4)

Pineapple, 1 ½ c cubed *fresh or frozen* (D4)

Bananas, 5 *ripe* (D4 & 6)

Red Delicious Apples, 5 c chopped, *approx. 3 apples* (D5)

Blueberries, 3 c *fresh or frozen* (D6)

Cherries, 2 c pitted, *fresh or frozen* (D7)

DAY ONE

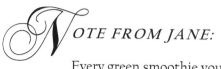

NOTE FROM JANE:

Every green smoothie you make is not only healthful, it's action, execution and fulfillment. The important thing is to build consistency. Drink more greens. Eat more greens. Think food abundance. We're adding to your food choices, not taking away.

You are here to create the habit of drinking your greens, absorbing it into your lifestyle as easily as the chlorophyll in green smoothies absorbs into your bloodstream.

We brush our teeth every day. Why? Because we know the alternative. That's how I think about my greens. I know the alternative is feeling thirsty, full and uninspired, with the nagging feeling that although I'm busy and working hard, it's dark in here and I want light.

I get that light by drinking my greens. That's why I want to help you make consuming green smoothies, like brushing your teeth, a habit.

Think about the outcome, what it feels like when you have more energy, what it feels like to accomplish a task in the pursuit of your dream. You have a higher self and you're capable of serving it. Drink your greens to achieve your dreams, one chlorophyll molecule at a time.

THOUGHT OF THE DAY:

I love beginnings.

I am capable of middles.

I rejoice in results.

WHO KNEW? GREEN SMOOTHIE

MAKES 3 ¾ CUPS OR 30 OUNCES

1 Tomato – *250g or 9 oz*

1 Cucumber, cut into 4 pieces – *240g or 8 oz*

½ head Iceberg Lettuce – *200g or 7 oz*

¼ t Sea Salt *optional*

Add the ingredients to your blender in the order listed, blend smooth, approximately 45 seconds. Pour into your favorite glass and savor.

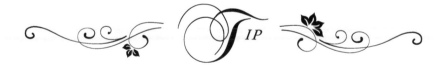

TIP

To receive optimal nutrition from green smoothies, they are best consumed alone in the mornings, so as not to compete with other foods you may be digesting.

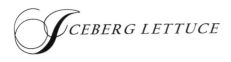CEBERG LETTUCE

Iceberg lettuce is not devoid of nutrition. Who knew? I investigated and found out it's a contender. Immediate promotion from garnish to main course. All my life I've heard that Iceberg lettuce has no nutrition in it, just pass it up for the darker greens, don't bother with it. So I thought, "Lettuce find out what is true about Iceberg lettuce."

Iceberg lettuce is high in water and for every 100 grams you sip, there is 95.64 grams of naturally filtered water and .90 grams of protein. Who knew Iceberg lettuce would have protein in it?

It also has Calcium, Iron, Vitamin A, Vitamin C, Thiamin, Potassium, B6, various amino acids, a low sodium content of 10mg and only 14 calories. It's good to know that Iceberg lettuce has value and that I can add it to my green smoothie rotation.

Iceberg lettuce is great for beginners, because if you're not ready to get into your deep, dark greens, this is a great way to start with a mild tasting, low glycemic green smoothie.

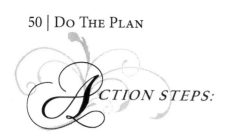

*A*CTION STEPS:

1. Recite today's affirmation aloud three times:

I am alive and feeling good.

I am alive and feeling good.

I am alive and feeling good.

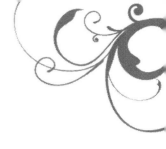

2. Smile.

Day Two

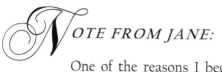

OTE FROM JANE:

One of the reasons I began drinking my greens is because I wanted to feel better. I know I'll never be or look 18 again but I wanted to feel 18 again with the hope and energy that comes with youth.

I've gotten pretty close. I feel positive and energetic and if that isn't reason enough to drink your greens, then I don't know what is.

Putting the emphasis on building your inner life takes pressure off of you and contributes to knowing your real worth and value as a human being. Yes, we all want to look good, but looking good can't cover for being unhappy or feeling useless. The beautiful thing is, when you feel good you do good and radiate beauty. Feeling good makes everyone beautiful.

It is not a straight line and it isn't always easy and you will have fits and starts and good days and bad. Congratulations, you're imperfect!

THOUGHT OF THE DAY:

I can stop taking myself so seriously.

I am capable of having fun and feeling joy.

Feel Better Green Smoothie

Makes 4 ½ cups or 36 ounces

4 c Apple Juice, fresh

2–3 leaves Lacinato/Dinosaur Kale – *100g or 3.5 oz substitute any variety kale*

½ t Cinnamon

2 T Lemon Juice, fresh

Add the ingredients to your blender in the order listed, blend smooth, approximately 45 seconds. Pour into your favorite glass and savor.

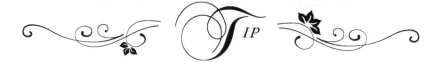

Tip

Peel fruit if not organic or pesticide free. Keep tender stems on parsley, cilantro, lettuces. Remove tough stems on kale, chard, collards.

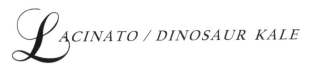 ACINATO / DINOSAUR KALE

I was craving a deep green smoothie and was captivated by a bowl of sunny yellow lemons on my kitchen counter. I combined the deep blue green of Lacinato/Dinosaur kale, fresh apple juice, a couple shakes of cinnamon and the juice of ½ lemon and it came out fantastic.

You can taste the kale, it's the foundation flavor. Then there's a little sweet from the apple juice. The cinnamon makes you think you're drinking dessert, and the lemon tops it off with an exclamation point, helping you feel better inside and out.

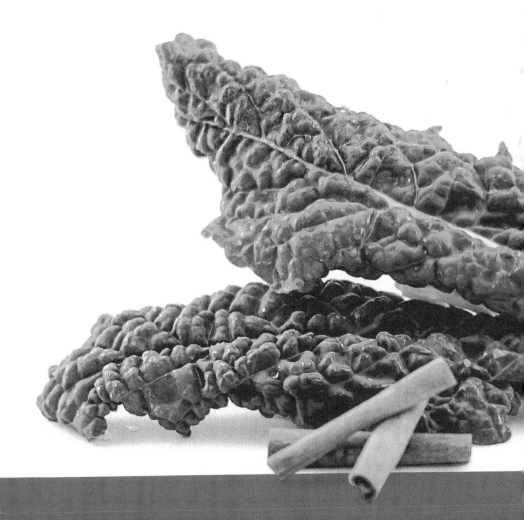

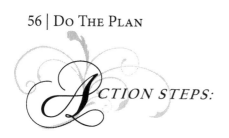

CTION STEPS:

1. Recite today's affirmation aloud three times:

    I am kind to me, too.

    I am kind to me, too.

    I am kind to me, too.

2. Find a section or drawer in your refrigerator that you can dedicate to your greens.

Clean it up so it shines. Taking the time to make this space in your refrigerator, harbinger of food emotions from distress to euphoria, is an important step in your commitment to these four weeks and beyond.

Day Three

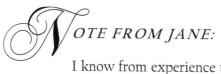

OTE FROM JANE:

I know from experience that if you drink your greens you will find the portal. I don't know when, but I do know why.

Drinking your greens is like compound interest. It may start out slowly, taking months or years to get some muscle, but then the amount begins to double and grow and double again and then double again and one day you have a nest egg from which comes great peace of mind.

Drinking your greens is similar. It takes time, but while that time is passing, there is activity inside of your body and mind. I can't know the specifics of what will happen to you, but I can share parts of what's happening to me, which I do throughout **Green Smoothie Habit**.

The drinking your greens journey is much like life itself, full of surprises, silences, shouts, serenity, activity, passivity and all kinds of twists and turns subtle and blunt, noticed and unnoticed. And then you get a knock on your green smoothie door and progress is delivering you flowers.

So have faith in the process of green smoothie drinking and Mother Nature. Let the greens work their chlorophyll and oxygen wonder. Let the fiber sweep you clean. Let the water plump your skin and outlook.

THOUGHT OF THE DAY:

'Please change' is one of the messages sent by physical and emotional discomfort.

Beautiful Skin Green Smoothie

Makes 4 ¼ cups or 34 ounces

1 Ruby Red Grapefruit, remove peel, pith, skin and
seeds – *500g or 18 oz*
substitute 2 oranges if you don't like grapefruit

1 Cucumber, cut into 4 pieces – *250g or 9 oz*

¾ bunch Parsley, fresh – *80g or 3 oz*
substitute any variety parsley

1 handful Mint, fresh – *22g or ¾ oz*

Add the ingredients to your blender in the order listed, blend smooth, approximately 45 seconds. Pour into your favorite glass and savor.

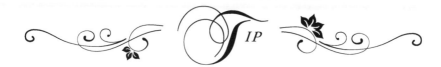

Wear ear protection if your blender is loud. Blend in the garage or basement if it's early morning or late evening and others are sleeping.

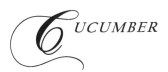UCUMBER

As we age our skin doesn't spring back the way it used to, but what we can do to help ourselves along is consume silica, a trace mineral that strengthens the body's connective tissues and is vital for healthy, elastic skin. The secret skin ingredient in this blend is silica rich cucumber, easy to enjoy in green smoothies.

The naturally distilled and purified water in these ingredients helps hydrate our skin from within and the tart grapefruit delivers an astringent, cleansing quality.

Remember, you don't have to be a vegetarian to enjoy green smoothies. I'm not, but by adding green smoothies to my diet, everything is better.

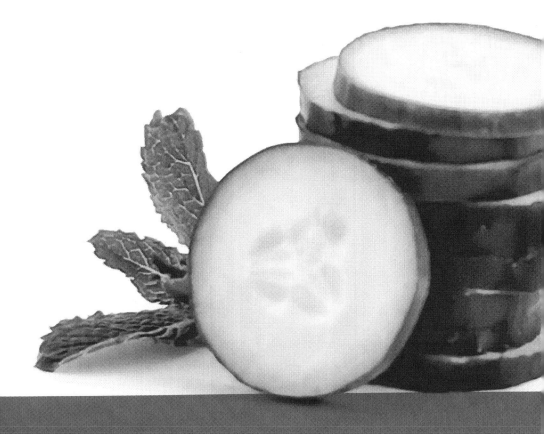

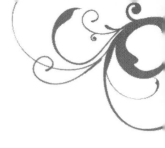

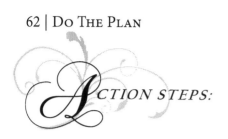

CTION STEPS:

1. Recite today's affirmation aloud three times:

I am strong.

I am strong.

I am strong.

2. Write why you want to drink your greens.

DAY FOUR

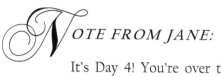

OTE FROM JANE:

It's Day 4! You're over the three day hump, congratulations! Now we can get some work done.

It took me decades to understand that my attitude is a physical choice, not an emotional one. Huh? The physical choice comes first and the emotional reward follows. Try it now, you'll see. Frown (physical) and you begin to feel bad (emotional). Smile (physical) and you feel better (emotional).

It's the same with choosing to blend fresh greens, capturing the chlorophyll and oxygen in a smooth, blood enriching liquid that is absorbed seamlessly through your intestinal walls, nourishing your lumen. Beyond the physical, this confluence of healthy blood and glowing light in your belly provides you, in my experience, with a lighted portal to your purpose.

As you go through these four weeks, smiling and sipping, I want you to dig deep and truly commit to completing **Green Smoothie Habit**.

THOUGHT OF THE DAY:

What is the alternative to drinking my greens?

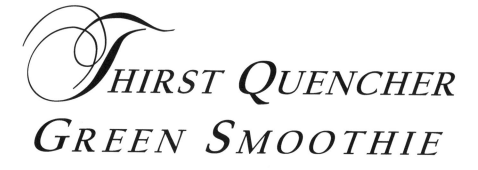

THIRST QUENCHER GREEN SMOOTHIE

MAKES 4 CUPS OR 32 OUNCES

> 1 c Water
>
> ½ c Orange Juice, fresh
>
> 1 ½ c Pineapple, cubed, fresh or frozen
>
> 4–6 leaves Romaine Lettuce – *100g or 3.5 oz*
>
> 1 Banana, ripe, fresh or frozen

Add the ingredients to your blender in the order listed, blend smooth, approximately 45 seconds. Pour into your favorite glass and savor.

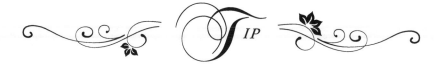

TIP

To freeze bananas, place ripe, peeled bananas into a freezer bag and they will keep for a couple of weeks. Make sure the peels have the brown sugar spots on them as this means they are at the peak of their ripeness, nutrition and flavor.

ROMAINE LETTUCE
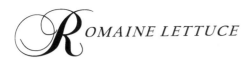

Listen to the crunch of the Romaine lettuce. That's freshness and goodness and chlorophyll and oxygen. Mmm, freshness, freshness.

When you get used to drinking your greens and getting all that high water content food in you, you feel less thirsty, and eating your water is something you begin to crave.

Many times we mistake thirst for hunger. Green smoothies, being a drink and a food, can satisfy both.

Drink your thirst quenching greens. Cheers!

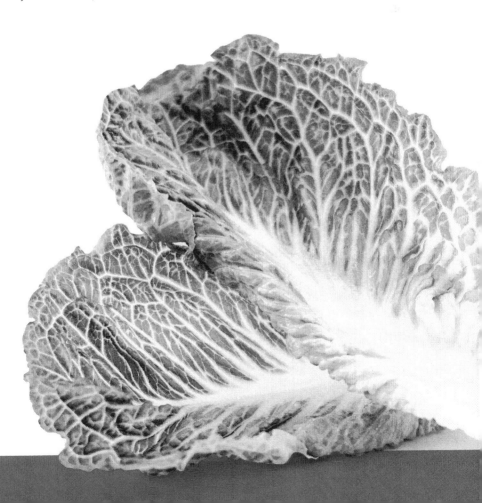

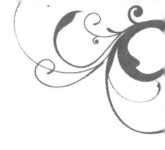

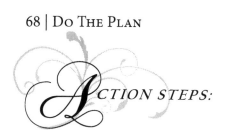

CTION STEPS:

1. Recite today's affirmation aloud three times:

   I am relaxed and safe.

   I am relaxed and safe.

   I am relaxed and safe.

2. Close your eyes, place one hand on your diaphragm (just above your belly button and below your ribs) and the other hand on your chest.

> Keeping your chest still, slowly inhale through your nose to the count of 4, filling your diaphragm. Exhale through your mouth to the count of 6, emptying your diaphragm. Do this 3 times.

DAY FIVE

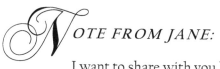*OTE FROM JANE:*

I want to share with you how I clean my blender. You can apply this information to any blender. (One of the reasons I use a Vitamix is because I don't have to take it apart to clean it.)

Level 1

Most of the time all I do to clean it is rinse it out and turn it upside down so that water doesn't seep beneath the gasket.

Level 2

Squirt 2 drops of dishwashing detergent into the blender container, fill it ⅔ with warm water, secure the lid and turn the blender on high for one minute. Your blender just became its own dishwasher. Rinse well, dry thoroughly.

Level 3

When you've owned your blender for a long time the container can become cloudy. Fill the container with water and a cup of vinegar, let it sit for three hours, then repeat the process and wipe down the inside of the container with a sponge. Consult your owner's manual to make sure you can use vinegar in your blender container.

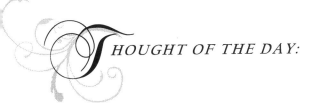

I am an effective self manager.

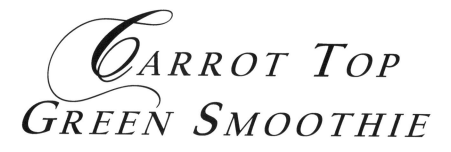

CARROT TOP GREEN SMOOTHIE

Makes 4 ¾ cups or 38 ounces

1 c Water

5 c Red Delicious Apples, cubed (about 3 apples)

1 handful Carrot Tops/Greens – *28g or 1 oz*

1 handful Mint, fresh – *22g or ¾ oz*

½ c Ice

Add the ingredients to your blender in the order listed, blend smooth, approximately 45 seconds. Pour into your favorite glass and savor.

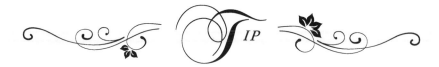

Fruits with insoluble fiber, such as apples, grapes and tomatoes may cause foam. To leave foam behind in the blender, pour out smoothie slowly from under the foam. Discard or compost foam.

CARROT TOPS / GREENS

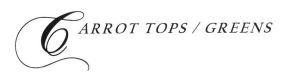

No need to throw out your carrot tops anymore. Break the cellular walls of carrot greens in your blender and drink up the lung protecting goodness. Carrot greens are packed with Vitamin A for our day and night vision and are an outstanding source of chlorophyll.

The mint complements the carrot greens, which by themselves are ho–hum, but when mixed with apples and mint we have something. Check out the color. Not so green, is it? All green smoothies are not green, but all green smoothies have greens in them.

It's light and fluffy in texture and there are little bits of red in it from the Red Delicious apple skins. Swoon with pleasure and surprise at how good carrot greens can taste.

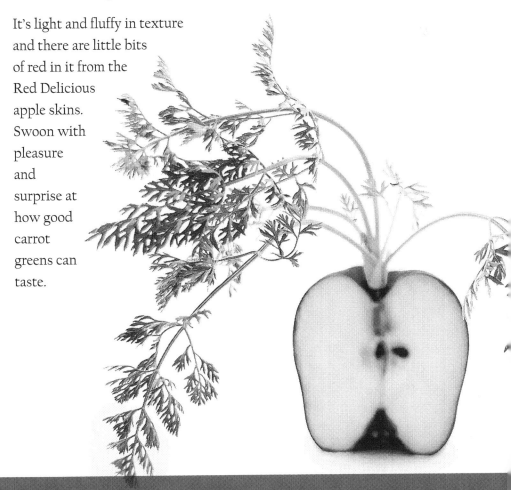

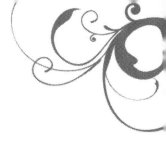

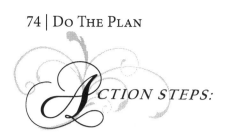

Action steps:

1. Recite today's affirmation aloud three times:

   I am taking action and it feels good.

   I am taking action and it feels good.

   I am taking action and it feels good.

2. Love your blender today.

Give the container a Level 3 treatment and wipe away spills or grime on and under your blender base. Take a soft toothbrush to the nooks and crannies.

DAY SIX

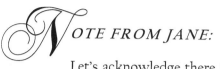

NOTE FROM JANE:

Let's acknowledge there is never a shortage of beginnings, but usually a shortage of finishing. Let's not let that happen with drinking our greens.

Quietly, consistently, persistently, let's drink our greens. Let's handle the loneliness and find the courage to finish, even if it's just this 28 days of **Green Smoothie Habit**.

I want for you to nourish the courage to finish by drinking your greens at home, at work, at play. Develop your inner strength by keeping your dream foremost in your mind. Work in the dark and the cold knowing that the light of your lumen flowing through your surface can keep you warm.

THOUGHT OF THE DAY:

I am not embarrassed to take my green smoothies to work, play and to the office for the day.

Or am I?

_____

_____

_____

_____

_____

_____

_____

_____

_____

_____

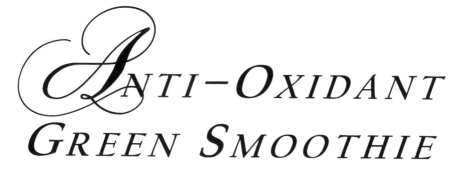

Anti-Oxidant Green Smoothie

MAKES 7 CUPS OR 56 OUNCES

1 c **Water**

3 c **Blueberries,** fresh or frozen

2–3 leaves **Collard Greens,** stems removed – *100g or 3.5 oz*

4 **Bananas,** ripe, fresh or frozen

2 c **Ice** *optional*

Add the ingredients to your blender in the order listed, blend smooth, approximately 45 seconds. Pour into your favorite glass and savor.

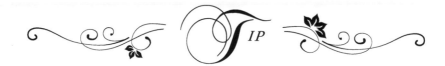

Tip

A thermos, cooler, glass water bottle or jar all work well for transporting green smoothies.

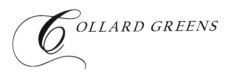OLLARD GREENS

This is a green smoothie filled with anti-oxidant rich blueberries and Vitamin K rich collard greens. Blueberries help to reduce the oxidative stress on our cells and Vitamin K helps us maintain healthy blood clotting and keeps blood vessels from calcifying.

This anti-oxidant elixir also helps support our anti-inflammatory systems and it tastes fantastic. There's enough here to share with family or friends and is thick enough to eat with a spoon, yet it can still be sipped through a straw. Kids love it.

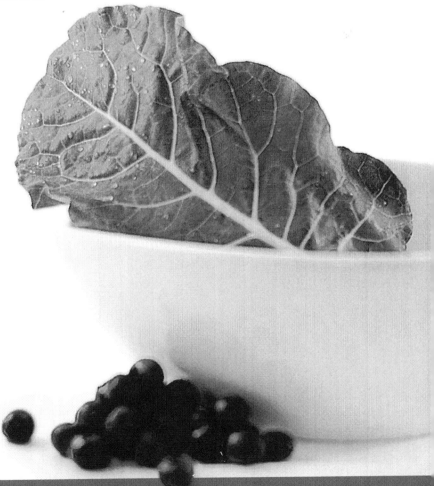

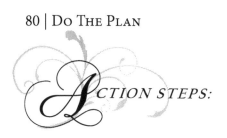
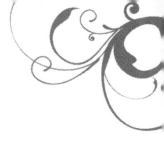

ACTION STEPS:

1. Recite today's affirmation aloud three times:

    I am worth taking care of.

    I am worth taking care of.

    I am worth taking care of.

2. Take time now and plan how you're going to transport your green smoothies and keep them cold. Now you are prepared to succeed.

_____

_____

_____

_____

_____

_____

_____

_____

_____

_____

DAY SEVEN

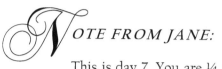

OTE FROM JANE:

This is day 7. You are ¼ of the way through **Green Smoothie Habit**: Drink Your Greens To Achieve Your Dreams. You are building the good and positive habit of drinking your greens.

Let's Recap

Have you been drinking your greens daily?	Yes	No
Are you doing your daily action steps?	Yes	No
Have you been contemplating the daily thoughts and repeating the affirmations?	Yes	No

If you circled YES three times, I am nodding approval. If you circled YES to drinking your greens and nothing else, you're in the game. If you haven't done anything yet, you're here, reading, so you still want in.

No matter where you are in your greens drinking, perhaps the lure of the portal is fading. Perhaps you feel alone and unsupported, no longer motivated or wondering what you thought all the fuss was about. I know how you feel, I have been there many times over many projects, intentions, promises and dreams.

Now is when you must breathe deeply and drink your greens whether you want to or not. Now is the time for positive self talk and action.

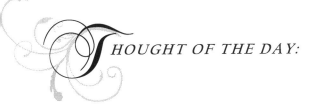

THOUGHT OF THE DAY:

I am gaining an understanding of my lumen, which is my inner light flowing through my surface.

#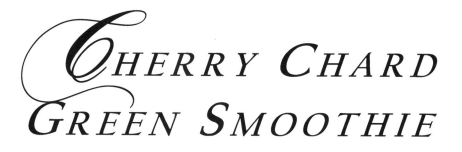

CHERRY CHARD
GREEN SMOOTHIE

MAKES 4 ½ CUPS OR 36 OUNCES

> 1 ½ c Water
>
> 2 c **Cherries,** pitted, fresh or frozen
>
> 2–3 leaves **Chard,** cut off bottom stems – *100g or 3.5 oz*
>
> 2 c Ice

Add the ingredients to your blender in the order listed, blend smooth, approximately 45 seconds. Pour into your favorite glass and savor.

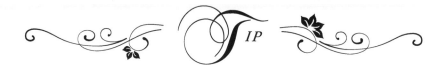

When using fresh fruit in your smoothies, make sure it is ripe or you won't get a delicious or nutritious result.

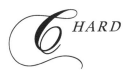

CHARD

I like this blend because it's not too sweet and is cool and refreshing, with the texture of a milkshake. I can taste a touch of the salty chard, which is high in bio-available organic sodium and calcium for strong bones and teeth.

Fresh cherries are delicious, nutritious, low in calories at 87 per cup and low on the Glycemic Index Scale at 22, good news if you are concerned about blood sugar levels.

You can further rotate your greens by choosing different varieties within the chard family, such as Swiss, Rainbow or Rhubarb chard, distinguished by their vibrant red, white or gold stems.

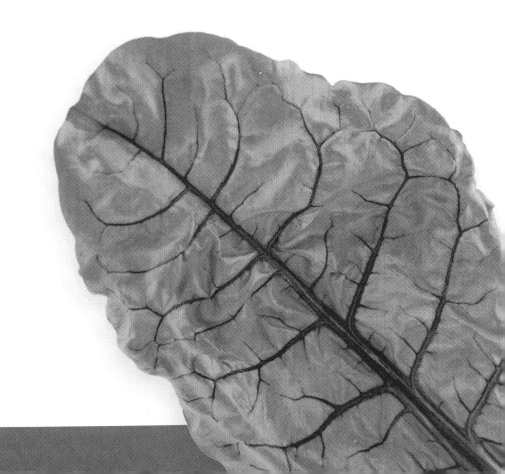

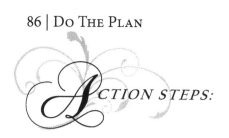

ACTION STEPS:

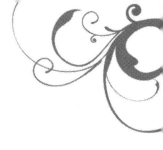

1. Recite today's affirmation aloud three times:

   I am confident and capable.

   I am confident and capable.

   I am confident and capable.

2. Write down a choice you recently made that gave you unsatisfactory results. You are not limited to food choices, it can be any area of your life.

Cross it out and write down what you could have done that would have given you a better outcome.

My Lumen

Check the box that best describes your lumen now:

Daily Greens Consumed		Lumen Forecast	
	Prepare for Planetary Travel		☐
	Sunny Inside and Out		☐
	Partially Sunny		☐
	Cloudy		☐
	Darkness		☐

~400g | ~200g | ~100g | ~50g

On to week two,

here we go...

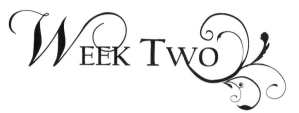 WEEK TWO

"I don't have to do everything the hard way and I don't have to have all the answers."

-Jane

Emotions are constantly moving, hence e-motion.

Instead of trying to pin them down, control or conquer them, let's go with them. Feeling blue? Drink your greens. Feeling on top of the world? Drink your greens. Confused? Drink your greens. Afraid? Drink your greens. Sick and tired? Drink your greens. Dreams comatose? Drink your greens.

Manage yourself by releasing family and friends from your expectations hook. It will be a huge relief to you and them. Nobody but you will know you're doing it, but everyone will feel better.

Fill the void with drinking your greens and working on your dream. Enjoy your forward motion.

WELCOME TO WEEK 2

By doing a 28 day intensive like this, we put ourselves under pressure to perform. Under that pressure, our weaknesses, areas of need, cracks and crevices of self doubt are more apt to surface, which is a good thing, because then we can identify them. We can fill them with green smoothies and let the mending begin.

Your greening journey will evolve, adapt, improve, rest, soar ahead, and take a back seat as the months and years roll on, but the consistent habit that you build here will always be with you.

Progress can be hard to measure, because sometimes it happens in areas that we are not focused on. While we're trying to lose weight and are concentrating on the way we look, the greens are building our inner strength and improving our mental and emotional poise. This poise can manifest itself in surprising new ways.

Progress is not a straight line, so don't fret when you find yourself going backwards or in circles. Work to accept the sharp turns, odd angles and dips and lifts that are the fun of being imperfect. Keep sipping your greens and eventually you'll arrive. That's progress.

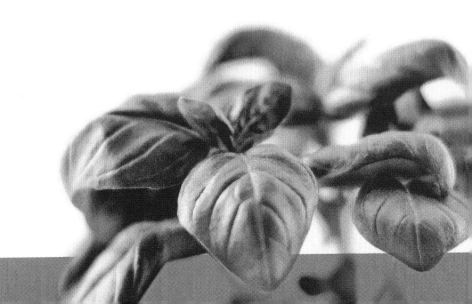

Menu & Shopping List

Day 8:	Easy Spinach Green Smoothie
Day 9:	Well Being Green Smoothie
Day 10:	Bok Choy Cheer Green Smoothie
Day 11:	Watercress Zing Green Smoothie
Day 12:	Dandelion Eyes Green Smoothie
Day 13:	Good Mood Green Smoothie
Day 14:	Papaya Basil Green Smoothie

GREENS & VEGGIES

Spinach, ½ bunch (D8)

Beet Greens, 1 bunch (D9)

Bok Choy, 2 leaves or 1 bunch Baby Bok Choy (D10)

Mint, 3 sprigs *fresh* (D10)

Watercress, 1 c (D11)

Dandelion, 4 leaves (D12)

Dill, ¼ c *fresh* (D13)

Basil, ¼ c *fresh* (D14)

FRUIT

Green Grapes, 4 c (D8)

Red Grapes, 4 c (D9)

Tangerine Juice, 3 c (D10)

Cucumber, 2 (D11, D13)

Lemon Juice, 1 T *fresh* (D11)

Oranges, 4 (D12)

Medjool Dates, 2 (D13)

Papaya, 3 c (D14)

Lime Juice, 1 t *fresh* (D14)

PANTRY

Flax Seed, 1 T *ground* (D9)

Sea Salt, ½ t *(optional)* (D11)

(D8 = Day 8, etc.) Use this key to help if you shop more than once a week.

DAY EIGHT

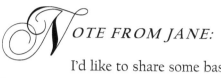

OTE FROM JANE:

I'd like to share some basic information about food combining because it helps us see our fruits and greens in relation to our digestive functions.

When you are making a green smoothie, you can relax knowing that your stomach acids can handle greens mixed with fruit. Why? Because leafy greens, unlike vegetables, are not a starch. They combine with fruit and do not need competing gastric juices for digestion. You can mix greens with melons, too. Usually it's best to eat melons alone, but it is my experience they blend well with leafy greens.

Pay attention to your body's digestive signals when consuming green smoothies. Sip slowly and chew your green smoothies so they mix with the salivary juices in your mouth. If a particular combination bothers you, eliminate it. There are endless green smoothie combinations. Find the ones that work for you, always remembering to rotate your greens, consuming as wide a variety as you can.

For best digestion, keep your green smoothies simple: fruit, greens, water.

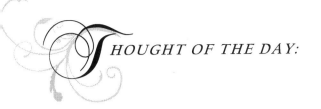

HOUGHT OF THE DAY:

Know what is true for you.

Easy Spinach Green Smoothie

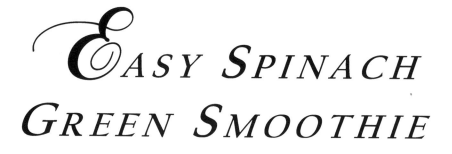

Makes 5 cups or 40 ounces

4 c Green Grapes, sweet

½ bunch Spinach – *100g or 3.5 oz*

2 c Ice

Add the ingredients to your blender in the order listed, blend smooth, approximately 45 seconds. Pour into your favorite glass and savor.

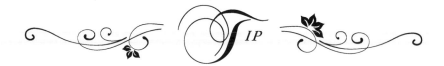

Starchy vegetables such as beets, carrots, zucchini, broccoli, etc., are not ideal for green smoothies due to their starch content, as starches and fruits require competing gastric juices for digestion.

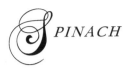PINACH

This yummy concoction tastes like white grape juice over crushed ice. It's cool, creamy, fortifying and freeing for your whole being.

I find that spinach builds not only muscle, but mental might and emotional fortitude. It may help prevent chronic fatigue, psoriasis, stroke, heart disease and cataracts. Spinach is mild in taste, an easy green to like and is available as tender, baby greens and bundled, mature leaves.

Let's fortify and free ourselves.

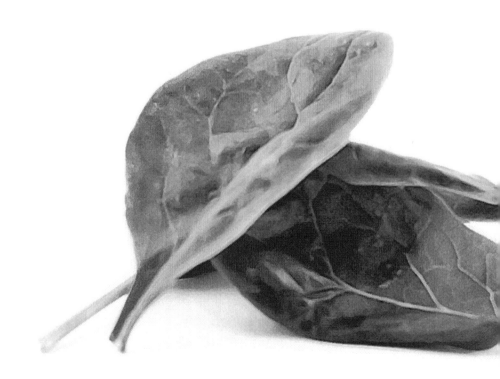

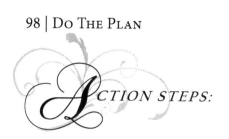
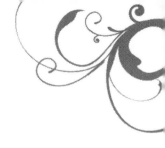

Action steps:

1. Recite today's affirmation aloud three times:

I am eating well.

I am eating well.

I am eating well.

2. List the leafy greens you can think of off the top of your head.

Take it with you the next time you shop and see what you missed. Add those missing greens to your list and rotate them in.

_____

_____

_____

_____

_____

_____

_____

_____

_____

_____

Day Nine

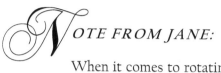OTE FROM JANE:

When it comes to rotating your greens, the ideal is 7 different greens in 7 days, as that gives you the wide variety you need to avoid alkaloid build-up and boredom, both necessary if you want to be in the green smoothie game long term.

In my local supermarket, there are 16 different greens and varieties thereof available on a regular basis. Lettuces, kales, spinach, chards, dandelion, carrot tops, parsleys, mints, beet greens, Bok Choy, turnip greens, mustard greens, cilantro, collards, dill, basil, etc. Then there are the natural food markets, small groceries, local farms and farmer's markets and of course, wild edible weeds, free for the picking if you know what you are doing and make sure you do, as some are poisonous.

Once you have been drinking your greens as long as I have, the need for them moderates. Whereas I used to drink half a gallon a day, the entire Vitamix container, sometimes I just don't need that much. Sometimes I do. Variety. Please do not become dogmatic about drinking your greens.

Listen to your body, not to me, and do what is best for yourself. You know.

THOUGHT OF THE DAY:

Display the kindness and
confidence that gets people to notice
you and wonder to themselves,

"Who's that?"

WELL BEING GREEN SMOOTHIE

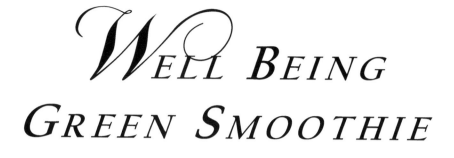

MAKES 4 ½ CUPS OR 36 OUNCES

4 c Red Grapes, sweet

1 bunch Beet Greens – *100g or 3.5 oz*

1 T Flax Seed, ground

2 c Ice

Add the ingredients to your blender in the order listed, blend smooth, approximately 45 seconds. Pour into your favorite glass and savor.

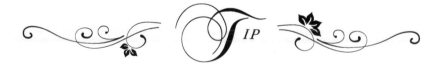

Green smoothies require no added fats or oils which can slow down absorption of nutrients. An exception is avocado, a fruit fat which works well in green smoothies, adding creaminess and satiety.

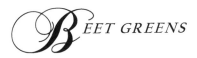 EET GREENS

Beet greens are rich in vitamins, minerals and carotenoids such as beta-carotene and lutein. Ground flax seed is wealthy with Omega-3's and fiber. "Put them together and what do you get? My colon is definitely not killing me yet."

The Well Being Green Smoothie helps prevent digestive tract syndromes and diseases by promoting healthy intestinal bacteria and encouraging regularity. It creates an overall sense of well being and relief and helps to clean and purify the alimentary canal.

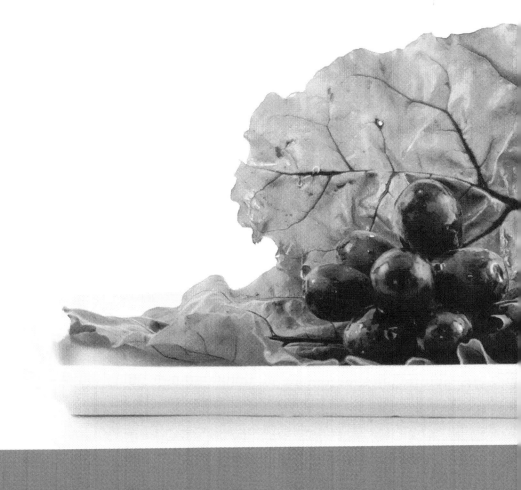

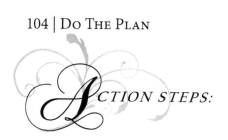

ACTION STEPS:

1. Recite today's affirmation aloud three times:

I am respecting my colon.

I am respecting my colon.

I am respecting my colon.

2. In the mission of mindfulness, before sipping your next green smoothie, bless it with the words "Thank you".

DAY TEN

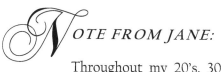OTE FROM JANE:

Throughout my 20's, 30's, 40's and now, I bounced around inside the walls of my life box of foods, plans, emotions, habits, desires, diets, fasting, this, that and the other thing, successfully keeping my weight where I wanted, but still enslaved by thinking about food all the time.

My food thoughts began evolving as I drank my greens regularly. Thanks to my greens hallelujah, food issues no longer drain my brain. When I first began drinking my greens, I couldn't get enough. I was starving inside for real nutrition and my body delighted in the flood of chlorophyll and oxygen I released into it.

I was changing. I could feel it. And not because I willed myself to change through diet, desire, or fear. The greens were changing me and there was nothing to be done about it, unless I stopped drinking my greens. I knew if I did, the mission would abort. It was scary at times. My newfound energy demanded work and action that I wasn't always sure I could deliver on.

Yet the thrill of being in a state of doing and not languishing in a state of wanting is an incredible pay off and I don't want to give it up. I continue to drink my greens, nourish my lumen and rejoice in the range of my lumen forecast; growing stronger, reaching further, shining brighter.

You can, too.

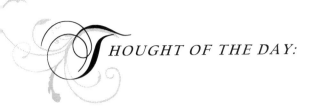

THOUGHT OF THE DAY:

Change takes courage.

Am I courageous?

_____

_____

_____

_____

_____

_____

_____

_____

_____

_____

_____

Bok Choy Cheer Green Smoothie

Makes 4 cups or 32 ounces

3 c Tangerine Juice, fresh squeezed

2–3 Bok Choy leaves or 1 bunch Baby Bok Choy – *100g or 3.5 oz*

2–3 sprigs Mint, fresh – *4g or 15 oz*

Add the ingredients to your blender in the order listed, blend smooth, approximately 45 seconds. Pour into your favorite glass and savor.

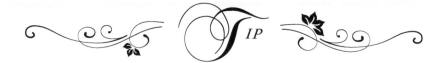

Tip

Try a glass straw through which to sip your green smoothies. It adds a mindful, elegant and timeless dimension to your sipping experience.

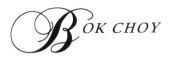 OK CHOY

My Bok Choy Cheer is a simple, refreshing elixir that introduces a new green to your rotation. Unique and delicious, Bok Choy is also known as Chinese cabbage in some locales.

Bok Choy is a cruciferous vegetable (use the leafy green tops of Bok Choy, not the white bulb) filled with Calcium, Iron, Vitamins A, C, D, Folate and anti-cancer compounds. Yes to blending and mending.

Baby Bok Choy is especially tender. The bulb isn't fully developed so you can use it whole in a green smoothie.

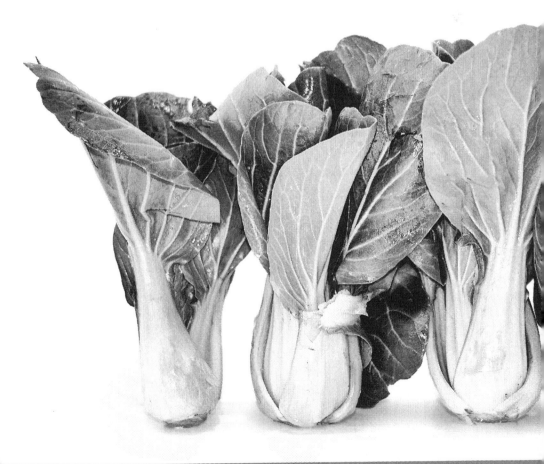

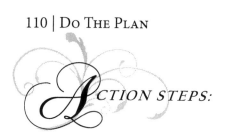

*A*CTION STEPS:

1. Recite today's affirmation aloud three times:

   I am enjoying leafy greens.

   I am enjoying leafy greens.

   I am enjoying leafy greens.

2. List the areas in your life in which you are fully convicted, that you will do even if you have to go it alone.

DAY ELEVEN

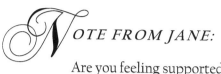OTE FROM JANE:

Are you feeling supported in your green smoothie habit? In your home, your kitchen, at work, with family and friends?

The tricky thing about feeling supported is that feelings of support follow the support structure we have in place. We have to create our own support structure. From my experience, nobody's going to create it for us.

The practical support comes in the form of your blender, your greens and fruits, your recipes, your kitchen layout, your refrigerator, your home and work schedule. Can you sit on your support? Is it strong enough to hold your weight?

The emotional support comes in the form of your expectations of yourself and others. We can't feel supported by someone if our expectations of them are unrealistic. They, like us, are imperfect.

That's why I trust this process of drinking my greens. I don't have expectations, I have trust. Subtle, but big difference. Be forewarned that switching out expectations for trust can leave a void, as trust has no agenda. Expectations do.

Your expectations of what you want to accomplish in this 28 days sets the stage for your success or failure. Yes, you have to think and dream big, but in order to accomplish those dreams, you have to act in small, incremental steps.

Get greening, stay greening, manage your expectations and choices and you will be a load bearing beam of support for yourself and others.

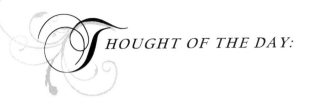

HOUGHT OF THE DAY:

My world supports my green smoothie habit and my green smoothie habit supports my world.

Watercress Zing Green Smoothie

Makes 2 cups or 16 ounces

1 c **Water**

1 **Cucumber**, cut into 4 pieces – *240g or 8 oz*

1 c **Watercress or Upland Cress** – *25g or 1oz*

1 T **Lemon Juice**, fresh

½ t **Sea Salt** *optional*

Add the ingredients to your blender in the order listed, blend smooth, approximately 45 seconds. Pour into your favorite glass and savor.

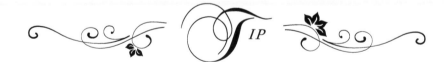

Tip

Remember to sip your green smoothies slowly and chew them, mixing them with your salivary juices before swallowing. Digestion begins in the mouth.

WATERCRESS

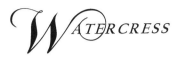

Watercress is bursting with phytonutrients, anti-oxidants, Calcium, Iron and Vitamins C and A. You can use Watercress and Upland Cress interchangeably in this blend.

It is wonderfully water rich and bursts in your mouth with a peppery, zingy flavor, livening up your savory green smoothie and clobbering cravings before they have a chance to creep in. Get ready to get zinged.

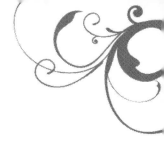

*A*CTION STEPS:

1. Recite today's affirmation aloud three times:

I am aware change is difficult,
but I can do it.

I am aware change is
difficult, but I can do it.

I am aware change is
difficult, but I can do it.

2. Name three people you can release from your expectations hook.

_____

_____

_____

_____

_____

_____

_____

_____

_____

_____

_____

DAY TWELVE

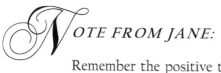*OTE FROM JANE:*

Remember the positive thought "I enjoy being patient" that I gave you in Chapter 4 Do The Plan, page 35?

"I enjoy being patient" works well when you are standing in a long line at the grocery store, are tired and hungry and want to get home. Those moments when you are most likely to think it matters not if you don't get your greens today.

"I enjoy being patient" also works well in the car when stuck in traffic, when dealing with people who upset you, and most of all when dealing with cravings.

"I enjoy being patient" is code for: I am in control of myself and understand the benefits of delayed gratification, which means waiting for a later, greater reward instead of indulging in a smaller, less enduring reward now.

I am happy I can provide you with an opportunity to enjoy being patient.

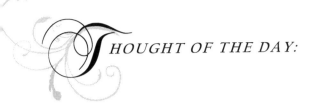

THOUGHT OF THE DAY:

We are our thoughts and actions.

_____

_____

_____

_____

_____

_____

_____

_____

_____

_____

DANDELION EYES GREEN SMOOTHIE

MAKES 3 CUPS OR 24 OUNCES

4 Oranges, sweet & juicy, peeled, remove seeds
 – 450g or 15 oz

4 leaves Dandelion *– 25g or 1 oz*

1 c Ice

Add the ingredients to your blender in the order listed, blend smooth, approximately 45 seconds. Pour into your favorite glass and savor.

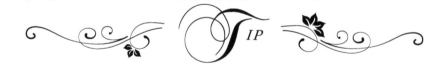

Adding citrus juice, especially lemon, to dandelion and kale helps to temper and neutralize their intense flavor profiles.

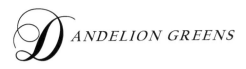

DANDELION GREENS

Even though dandelion is considered a 'bitter' green, this is a mild tasting smoothie with sweet citrus overtones.

Dandelion greens are beneficial for bone and liver health, diabetes, skin care, acne, weight loss, jaundice and anemia.

Dandelion greens contain beta carotene, Vitamins B1, B2, B5, B6, C and E and the minerals Iron, Potassium, Phosphorous, Magnesium and Zinc. Come on, who can say no to that?

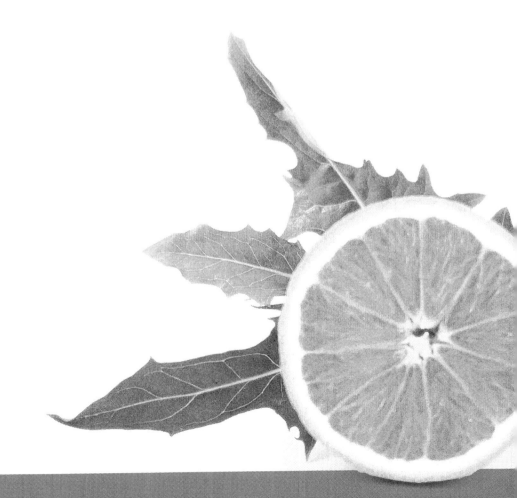

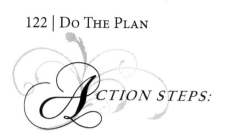

*A*CTION *STEPS:*

1. Recite today's affirmation aloud three times:

   I am valuable.

   I am valuable.

   I am valuable.

2. Record what you imagine your lumen looks and feels like:

Color, reach, purpose, temperature, strength, taste, texture, sound, opacity, transparency, etc.

DAY THIRTEEN

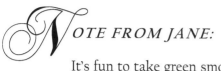

OTE FROM JANE:

It's fun to take green smoothies to work and play because you know how good you'll feel all day. Fresh, slim, and cheery. Can't beat the green smoothie good mood.

If going to the office, a thermos or cooler works great. If you have a refrigerator available at work, even better. By taking the time to create green smoothies and take them with you, you are going to sip the food you want to feel like, valuable, energetic, slimming and sumptuous. This guarantees you not just a great day at the office or with the kids, but an adventure in self worth and choices.

Yes, it takes effort to be prepared, but it's worth it. When I can, I take my green smoothies with me. Through long days of work or play and wanting to treat myself well, they have never let me down.

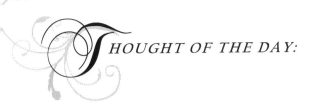

HOUGHT OF THE DAY:

Whatever and wherever you are now is really what and where you want to be or you would be someone else somewhere else.

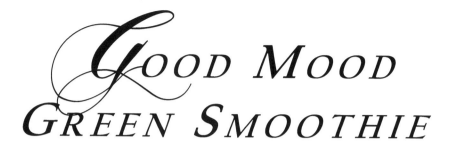

GOOD MOOD GREEN SMOOTHIE

MAKES 3 CUPS OR 24 OUNCES

2 c Water

1 Cucumber, cut into 4 pieces – *240g or 8 oz*

¼ c Dill, fresh, lightly packed – *15g or ½ oz*

2 Medjool Dates, pitted

Add the ingredients to your blender in the order listed, blend smooth, approximately 45 seconds. Pour into your favorite glass and savor.

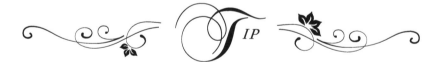

For your convenience, see page 264 in the Appendix for the Glycemic Index Scale listing of fruits used in Green Smoothie Habit.

DILL

I love the aroma and flavor of dill. It is full of anti-oxidants, phytonutrients and is a pungent and delicious herb. This blend has a hint of sweetness from the Medjool dates.

This is a deep, dark green drink that helps control cravings and energizes you without sugar spikes and I always feel so good on this blend. I hope you do, too.

If desired, dill can be replaced with the fresh herb of your choice, i.e., parsley, mint, cilantro, basil...

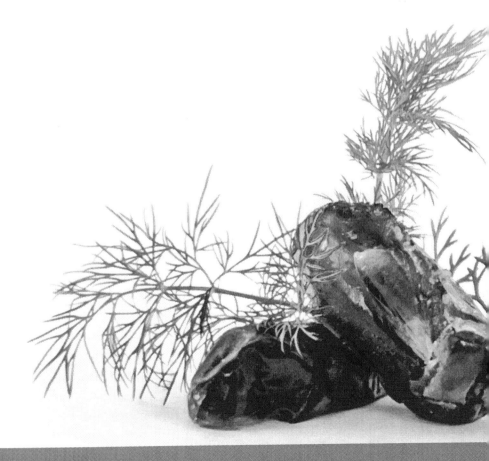

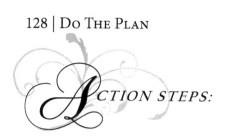

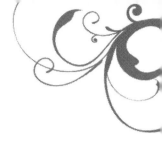

ACTION STEPS:

1. Recite today's affirmation aloud three times:

   I am drinking my greens.

   I am drinking my greens.

   I am drinking my greens.

2. You're feeling fresh, slim and cheerful. Name a choice you made that helped you achieve the green smoothie good mood.

DAY FOURTEEN

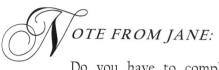

NOTE FROM JANE:

Do you have to complete **Green Smoothie Habit** in 28 consecutive days? I want you to, but I know that sometimes it isn't possible.

In my experience, there is the initial rush of being enthusiastic and committed and then a week or two into it real life sticks its head up and pushes you around.

The routine you imagined in your head is not feasible today or tomorrow due to a family or work change that you didn't foresee when you were in the initial glow.

All is not lost. You may have to miss a day. If you do, it's not the end of the world. **Green Smoothie Habit** is not going anywhere.

Think about drinking your greens as a lifestyle, so if something happens that causes you to miss a day, it's okay. Breathe and recite "I enjoy being patient".

Do whatever portion of the action steps you can for that day. It will keep you in the game and looking forward to your next green smoothie. Do what you can, which is better than quitting and doing nothing.

We are all imperfect, trying our best to live good lives and experience good work and health and the rewards that come along with them.

I reach out to you now and ask you to accept yourself as you are and move ahead imperfectly, move ahead as best you can and make do with what you have.

THOUGHT OF THE DAY:

I can choose the thoughts I dwell upon as I choose the foods I live on.

Papaya Basil Green Smoothie

Makes 3 cups or 24 ounces

3 c ripe **Papaya,** fresh

¼ c **Basil,** fresh – *10g or ½ oz*

1 t **Lime Juice,** fresh

1 c **Ice**

Add the ingredients to your blender in the order listed, blend smooth, approximately 45 seconds. Pour into your favorite glass and savor.

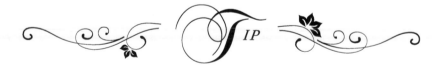

Tip

Kids like green smoothies, too. Make them sweet. Call them green monster drinks. Provide fun straws. Your kids won't know they're getting their greens, but you will.

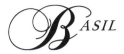

BASIL

Feel happy, hydrated and youthful sipping this luscious and light green smoothie. Ripe papaya and basil go together like green and smoothie. It has a pudding like texture. Eat with a spoon or sip through a straw.

Fresh basil is not just for pesto. It is a delicious and soothing herb known the world over for its tender, domed leaves, essential oils and food and eating pleasures.

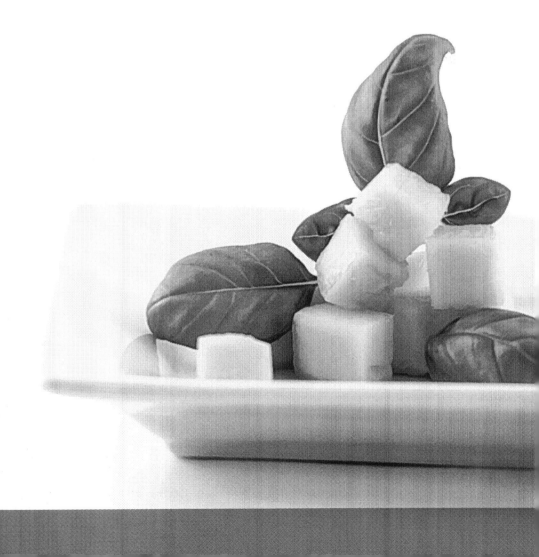

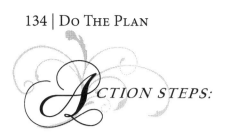

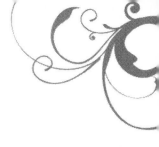

*A*CTION STEPS:

1. Recite today's affirmation aloud three times:

I am free to choose my attitude.

I am free to choose my attitude.

I am free to choose my attitude.

2. Plan a constructive response or solution in the event you are unable to complete Green Smoothie Habit in 28 consecutive days.

My Lumen

Check the box that best describes your lumen now:

Daily Greens Consumed	Lumen Forecast

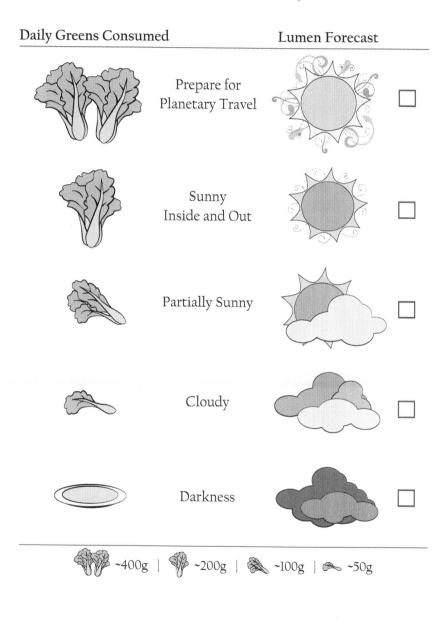

Prepare for
Planetary Travel ☐

Sunny
Inside and Out ☐

Partially Sunny ☐

Cloudy ☐

Darkness ☐

🥬 ~400g | 🥬 ~200g | 🥬 ~100g | 🥬 ~50g

On to week three,

here we go...

WEEK THREE

"I accept myself as I am."

-*Jane*

Green smoothie dreams can come true for you.

It's work, but what is the alternative? We either work on our own dreams or we work on someone else's.

Dreams don't have to be big. My greatest feelings of accomplishment come from achieving the small steps that are necessary to accomplish a goal.

I think you will be amazed at how your daily, positive actions add up to an appreciable accomplishment. You can be proud of yourself, and you can apply your ability to create the habit of drinking your greens to other aspects of your life. One sip, one step, one task, one action at a time we build our dream world.

Drink your greens, rotate your greens, enjoy your greens. Regardless of your present diet, which I am not concerned with, get your greens to achieve your dreams.

If the only ongoing change you make is to add a green smoothie to your morning routine, you are giving yourself a nutrient dense and delightful head start.

May you experience abundance in health, spirit, energy, truth and happiness. Be who you are abundantly and I see no reason why your green smoothie dreams can't come true.

WELCOME TO WEEK 3!

You are halfway to your Certificate of Achievement! You have made it through the first two weeks, are familiar with the routine and know what to expect as you continue building your green smoothie habit.

In this third week, you may lack some of the enthusiasm with which you started. Perhaps making daily green smoothies is beginning to resemble a chore.

That's okay, just take a deep breath and finish **Green Smoothie Habit** whether you want to or not. You don't need to be excited, you just need to do it. The next 14 days are going to pass whether you drink your greens or not, whether you do the action steps or not.

Just imagine the feeling of gratification and pride you will have when you finish. Not almost finish, but finish. Not perfectly finish, but finish.

Keep blending and sipping your greens. You will be glad you did.

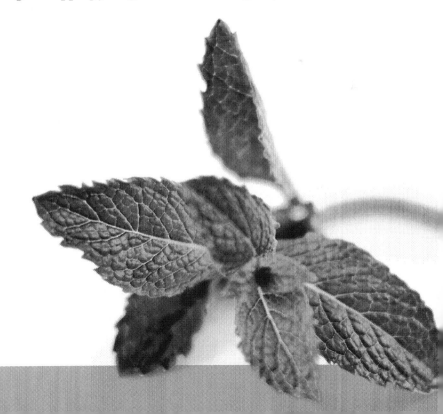

MENU & SHOPPING LIST

DAY 15:   Endless Endive Green Smoothie

DAY 16:   Kale Beauty Green Smoothie

DAY 17:   Quiet Time Green Smoothie

DAY 18:   Pear Party Green Smoothie

DAY 19:   Electrolyte Green Smoothie

DAY 20:   Potassium Power Green Smoothie

DAY 21:   Bright Morning Green Smoothie

GREENS & VEGGIES

Curly Endive, handful (D15)

Curly Kale, 3 leaves (D16)

Butter Head/Bibb Lettuce, 2 leaves (D17)

Mixed Baby Greens, 1 c (D18)

Celery, 2 stalks with leafy tips (D19)

Green Leaf Lettuce, 2 leaves (D20)

Spinach, 2 c (D21)

PANTRY

Sea Salt, ¼ t *optional*,(D19)

Black Pepper, pinch *ground* (D19)

FRUIT

Watermelon, 3 c (D15)

Lemon Juice, 1 t *fresh* (D15)

Grapes, Red 2 c (D16)

Mango, 2 c *fresh or frozen* (D16)

Nectarines, 2 c (D17)

Pears, 2 c (D18)

Tomatoes, Roma, 4 (D19)

Lime Juice, 1 T *fresh* (D19)

Bananas, 2 (D20)

Cucumber, 1 (D21)

Lemon, 1 (D21)

Medjool Dates, 3 (D21)

(D15 = Day 15, etc.) Use this key to help if you shop more than once a week.

Day Fifteen

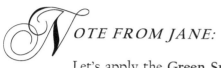OTE FROM JANE:

Let's apply the **Green Smoothie Habit** mindset to our whole lives, not just food. I want to share with you how I do it so you can do it, too.

For instance:

Physical

I am not an Olympic athlete, but I do know that exercise and physical culture appropriate to me improves my life.

Mental

I am not a psychiatrist, but I do know that I know the answers to my problems when I am brave enough to know I know.

Emotional

I am not a therapist but I do know that my emotions provide me with valuable information.

These are baselines, just like drinking my greens is a food consumption baseline. Think now about your physical, mental and emotional baselines. Your attention will soon begin to force some clarity from the fog.

I hope that these 28 days of drinking your greens begins a journey beyond food to a place where you are true to your whole being. That is the essence of **Green Smoothie Habit**.

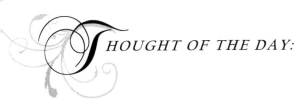

THOUGHT OF THE DAY:

I am clear in my choices
because I am calm
enough to choose clearly.

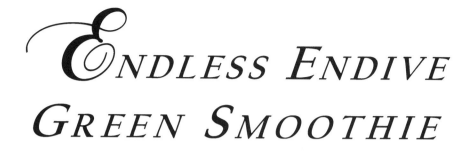

Endless Endive Green Smoothie

MAKES 2 1/4 CUPS OR 18 OUNCES

3 c Watermelon, remove rind and seeds

1 handful Curly Endive, also known as Frisée – *50g or 2 oz*

1 t Lemon Juice, fresh

Add the ingredients to your blender in the order listed, blend smooth, approximately 45 seconds. Pour into your favorite glass and savor.

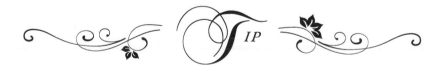

Walking and deep breathing increases our oxygen intake and complements our green smoothie habit, so head out for a 15 minute walk, breathe deeply and give thanks.

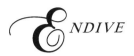 ENDIVE

My Endless Endive Green Smoothie is your personal bright and cheerful day delivery system. Watermelon, curly endive and a squeeze of lemon juice.

Endive is full of Folate and is an important nutrient for our mental strength and clarity, and it helps to ward off depression. So fill up your blender, endlessly, with Endive.

If curly endive is not available, substitute with spinach or collards as they are also high in Folate.

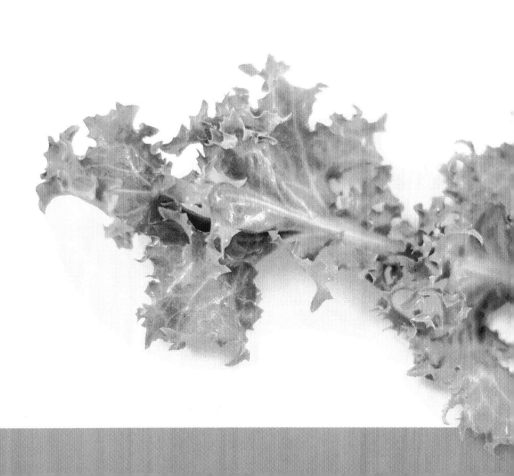

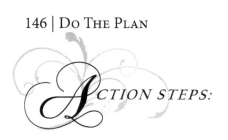

Action steps:

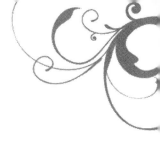

1. Recite today's affirmation aloud three times:

I am improving myself.

I am improving myself.

I am improving myself.

2. Complete the baseline sentences about yourself.

I am not an Olympic athlete, but I do know...

I am not a psychiatrist, but I do know...

I am not a therapist, but I do know...

Day Sixteen

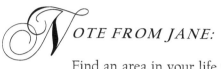

OTE FROM JANE:

Find an area in your life upon which you can improve. Maybe you want to clean your closets, weed your garden or paint your bathroom. Maybe you want to lose weight, change your look or throw out all your cosmetics and start fresh.

Maybe your changes must be monumental, switching careers, mates, cities. The important point to remember is that all change, big, medium or small, can only be accomplished one step at a time.

That's what I like about drinking my greens. One green at a time. One smoothie at a time. One sip at a time. You are creating a green smoothie habit to serve you, not the other way around. The point is not for you to become a slave to making green smoothies.

It's time to pioneer your dream. To pioneer is to be first, to look ahead and see what others cannot, won't or are not interested in seeing. Your dream is your responsibility. Do something. Take one small step forward in the accomplishment of your dream.

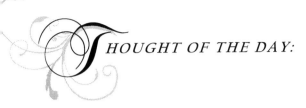

THOUGHT OF THE DAY:

Begin to dream.

KALE BEAUTY GREEN SMOOTHIE

MAKES 3 ½ CUPS OR 28 OUNCES

2 c **Red Grapes**

2 c **Mango,** fresh or frozen

3 leaves **Curly Kale** – *50g or 1 ½ oz*

1 c **Ice**

Add the ingredients to your blender in the order listed, blend smooth, approximately 45 seconds. Pour into your favorite glass and savor.

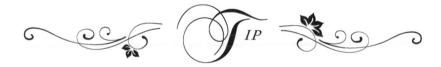

TIP

Gelatinous fruits such as mangoes, bananas, blueberries, peaches and pears contain soluble fiber which lend themselves to a creamy smoothie that doesn't separate.

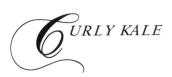URLY KALE

Do you want to feed your skin at the cellular level? I do, too. This smoothie is green kale, yellow mango and red grapes. Our phytonutrients (phyto is Greek for plant) are in these brightly colored foods.

My Kale Beauty Green Smoothie is sweet and deep green for super clean inside and out. The high water content of the kale, mango and grapes helps to plump up our skin and prevent dehydration and loss of elasticity. Hair, eyes and skin glow.

It is a vibrant color of green with purple specks from the grape's skins. It tastes fresh and full of life. You will feel beautiful.

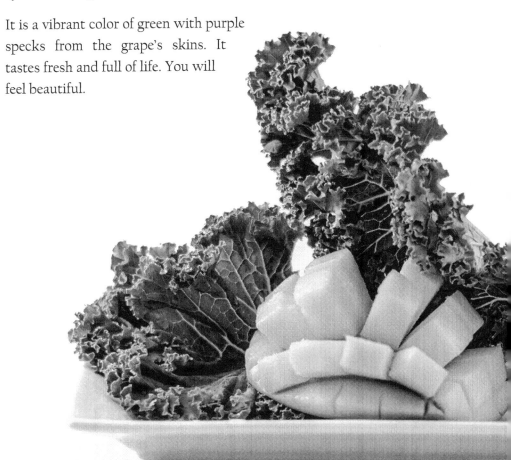

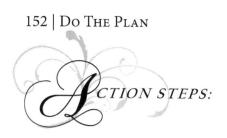

*A*CTION *STEPS:*

1. Recite today's affirmation aloud three times:

   I am glad I am nourishing my lumen.

   *I am glad I am
   nourishing my lumen.*

   *I am glad I am nourishing
   my lumen.*

2. What small step forward can you take in the direction you dream of heading? Be specific.

Day Seventeen

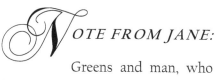

OTE FROM JANE:

Greens and man, who knew we had so much in common and could nourish each other?

It is never too late to create your own code, trust your mystery, respect your dreams and do it, do it, do it.

You are nourishing your lumen, the light of your oxygen breathing life. From your newborn squawk to now, you are alive, you are here, you matter.

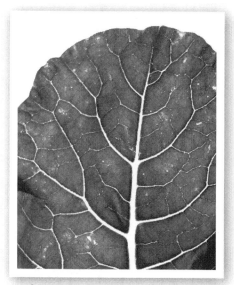

Leafy green vein network, rich in nutrients for nourishing blood and lumen.

The greens ignite you and hold your dreams out in front of you and say, "Come and get it." Do not be afraid of your energy and your dreams. They come in peace.

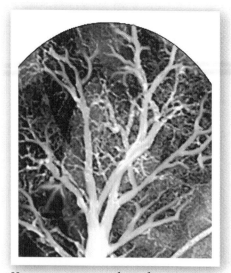

Human vein network, rich in nutrients extracted from green smoothies.

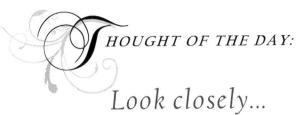

THOUGHT OF THE DAY:

Look closely...

...the vein networks in leafy greens resemble the vein networks in us.

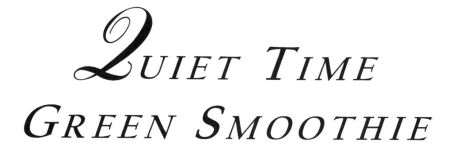QUIET TIME GREEN SMOOTHIE

Makes 2 ½ cups or 20 ounces

> 1 c Water
>
> 2 c Nectarines, ripe
>
> 2 leaves Butterhead/Bibb Lettuce – *25g or 1 oz*

Add the ingredients to your blender in the order listed, blend smooth, approximately 45 seconds. Pour into your favorite glass and savor.

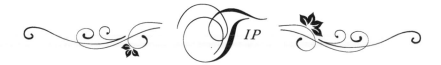

Our greens are only as nutritious as the soil in which they are grown. Make instant compost by diluting green smoothie remnants and pouring them in the garden.

BUTTERHEAD LETTUCE

This smoothie is just what you need when you want some quiet time. If you are thinking on a problem, letting it cure until the answer appears, savor this serene smoothie during the process.

Tender, organic Butterhead lettuce and sweet, ripe, juicy nectarines go together perfectly for a perfectly serene green smoothie.

Make sure the nectarines are ripe or you won't get the same result. Pour it into a pretty crystal glass. It is smooth as silk, and has little red flecks in it from the nectarine skin. It's beautiful inside and out, this glass of serenity.

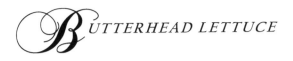

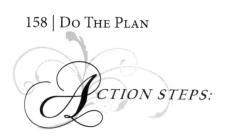

*A*CTION *STEPS:*

1. Recite today's affirmation aloud three times:

I am not afraid.

I am not afraid.

I am not afraid.

2. Choose a leaf from one of your greens to examine and think upon.

Write a poem about your leaf discovery.

DAY EIGHTEEN

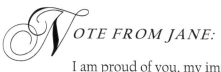OTE FROM JANE:

I am proud of you, my imperfect green smoothie baby bird. You are not so young anymore. You are out there flapping your wings and flying.

I am one of you. I open my refrigerator and put together green smoothies, just like you do. I use recipes as is or for inspiration, just like you do. I try new greens, make some winners and losers, just like you do.

I drink my greens and let the greens work their magic, just like you do. I put one foot in front of the other in the direction I dream of heading, just like you do.

I have fits and starts, stops and restarts, stalls, pauses, stumbles, breakdowns, pick ups, blunders, satisfactions, victories and ultimately progress, just like you do.

I enjoy it and I hope you do, too. Better to be imperfectly alive and doing, taking action and moving forward than to sit and want, never taking action. I am proud of us.

Please do not underestimate what you have to offer. I don't underestimate you. I know what you are going through and what it takes. I applaud and admire you.

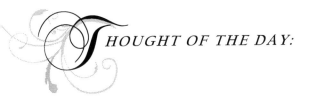

HOUGHT OF THE DAY:

*Finding green smoothie friends
is easy when you join MyHabit,
your free support community at*

GreenSmoothieHabit.com

Pear Party Green Smoothie

Makes 2 ½ cups or 20 ounces

1 c Water

2 c Pears, ripe

1 c Mixed Baby Greens – *25g or 1 oz*

Add the ingredients to your blender in the order listed, blend smooth, approximately 45 seconds. Pour into your favorite glass and savor.

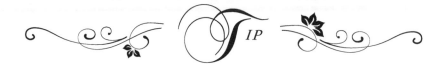

Tip

Show off your green smoothies in clear containers. The color is a great conversation starter and a surefire way to find other green smoothie people.

MIXED BABY GREENS

My Pear Party Green Smoothie combines sweet, juicy pears with mixed baby lettuces to deliver a delicate flavor and potent health properties.

Mixed baby lettuces are rich in chlorophyll, oxygen, water, Vitamin C, Vitamin A, Calcium and Iron, too. The pears are high in pectin, help nourish the macula and contain boron, which helps us retain calcium and prevent osteoporosis.

It's a green goodness pear party in a glass.

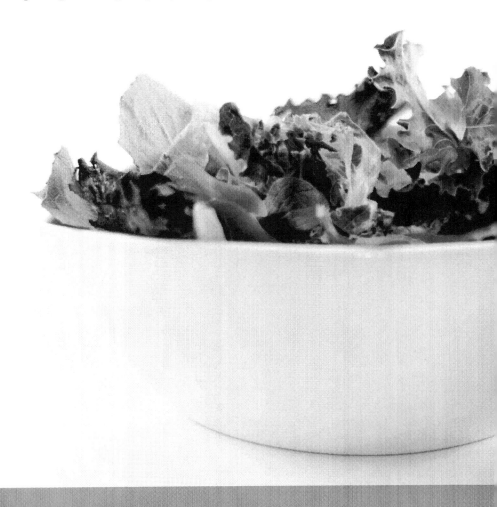

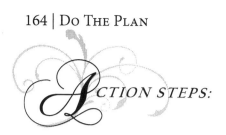

ACTION STEPS:

1. Recite today's affirmation aloud three times:

I am responsible for myself and I like it.

I am responsible for myself and I like it.

I am responsible for myself and I like it.

2. What are you passionate about, good at and can help others with?

I am passionate about

I am good at

I can help others with

Day Nineteen

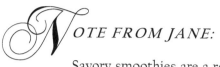TE FROM JANE:

Savory smoothies are a refreshing break from traditional green smoothies made with sweet fruit. Tomatoes, cucumbers, avocados, bell peppers and other vegetable-fruits are low on the Glycemic Index Scale of 1-100, coming in under 50, which is considered low glycemic.

Savory smoothies can help those of us who want to control our fruit sugar intake but still want our green smoothies. And they can help to quell the green smoothie craving monster, the one that sometimes pops up after sipping a high in fruit sugar green smoothie and gets you thinking you're hungry. It's happened with me. Low sugar savory smoothies help to solve that problem.

Another benefit to savory smoothies is that they surprise our taste buds with new flavors. It is important that you not only get a wide variety of greens, but that you get a wide variety of flavors, taste sensations and mouth feel.

You don't always have to make a blender full. A cucumber and sprig of parsley, voila!, a savory cocktail. Many savory green smoothies benefit from the addition of avocado for creaminess and lemon or lime for zing.

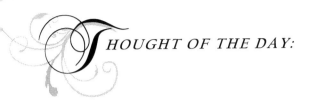

THOUGHT OF THE DAY:

Green smoothie making is an art and I have a picture to paint.

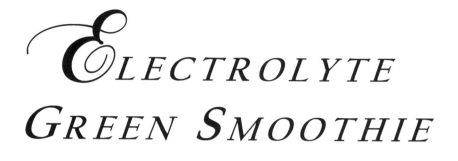

ELECTROLYTE GREEN SMOOTHIE

MAKES 2 CUPS OR 16 OUNCES

4 Roma/Plum Tomatoes – *350g or 12 oz*

2 stalks Celery, save the leafy tips for garnish – *115g or 4 oz*

1 T Lime Juice, fresh

¼ t Sea Salt *optional*

GARNISH:
  Pinch Black Pepper, fresh ground
  Celery Leaf Tips

Add the ingredients to your blender in the order listed, blend smooth, approximately 45 seconds. Pour into your favorite glass, garnish, and savor.

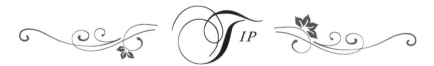

TIP

Remember that low glycemic, savory green smoothies are excellent choices for those of us concerned about blood sugar levels.

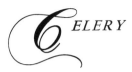

CELERY

Here is a savory smoothie that's a treat, but not sweet. A treat with a twist. I enjoy this refreshing cocktail. It's simple and elegant. Add water if you want a thinner texture.

Sometimes tomatoes get foamy when blended. If you don't like the fluffy texture, run the blender on low for 10 seconds or let your smoothie rest and after several minutes the foam reduces.

The lycopene in tomatoes acts as an anti-oxidant, neutralizing free radicals that can damage our cells. Celery is high in potassium and sodium, and when celery-based juices are consumed after a workout they serve as great electrolyte replacement drinks.

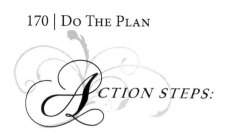

*A*CTION STEPS:

1. Recite today's affirmation aloud three times:

    I am creative.

    I am creative.

    I am creative.

2. Create a savory green smoothie that you can enjoy and add to your repertoire.

Try it now for a second smoothie, or try it when you're out of the nest.

DAY TWENTY

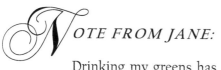OTE FROM JANE:

Drinking my greens has motivated me to cull, clean, organize and look at the physical items in my life with a new perspective, so that my outside world is as fresh and high vibration as my inside.

It is easier to accumulate things than to get rid of them, but I am doing it. I feel fabulous that I can now open my bedroom closet door and see my shoes and clothes without storage boxes and items that belong elsewhere.

Drinking my greens cleans me on the inside which spurs me to clean on the outside, to tidy up and prioritize my kitchen, my home, my life.

Clutter doesn't serve you, but serves to confuse you. Visual clutter can keep you from making your green smoothie in the morning if your blender is not accessible and ready to use or if you forgot you have greens because they are buried at the bottom of the refrigerator and you can't see them.

If I can't see it and I can't reach it, I don't want it. Make it a baseline: your see and reach kitchen, your see and reach closets.

Keep the aisles and shelves of your life clutter free and organized. Put your blender front and center, make room for more greens and they will waltz in.

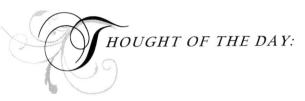

HOUGHT OF THE DAY:

Clutter makes it difficult to change, take advantage of new opportunities or welcome new experiences into your life.

Potassium Power Green Smoothie

Makes 3 cups or 24 ounces

1 c Water

2 Bananas, ripe, fresh or frozen – *240g or 8 oz*

2 leaves Green Leaf Lettuce – *50g or 2 oz*

1 c Ice

Add the ingredients to your blender in the order listed, blend smooth, approximately 45 seconds. Pour into your favorite glass and savor.

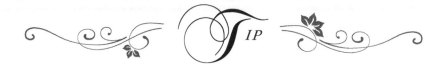

Tip

Visit a local, organic farm and buy greens from the source. Inquire about wild edible greens. Take the kids.

GREEN LEAF LETTUCE
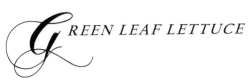

I created Potassium Power because I wanted a smoothie that would help me build my strength, inside and out. I looked to the great apes for inspiration and came up with bananas and green leaf lettuce.

The potassium in the bananas can help us regulate our blood pressure, our fluid levels and our muscle control, as if we were an engine. Get the great ape benefit of strength and power.

Remember the tip I gave you on day four: a properly ripened banana has brown spots on its peel, indicating the starch has converted to sugar and it is at the peak of its ripeness, flavor and nutrition.

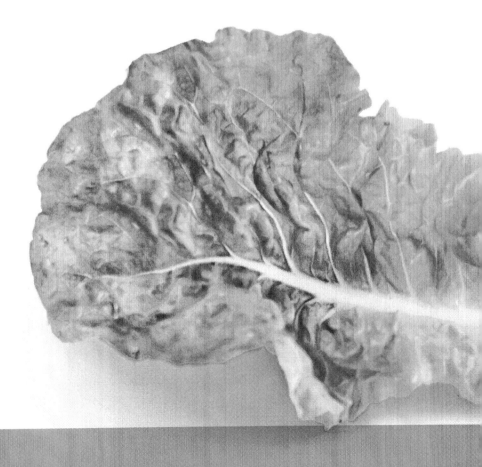

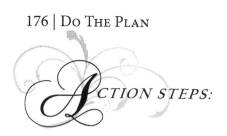

ACTION STEPS:

1. Recite today's affirmation aloud three times:

I am completing today's action steps.

I am completing today's action steps.

I am completing today's action steps.

2. Today, I will de-clutter, clean and organize the following specific area that is important to me.

Desktop, closet, car, drawer, etc.

DAY TWENTY-ONE

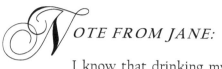

OTE FROM JANE:

I know that drinking my greens and treating myself like the valuable person I am has fed my inner life and contributed to the development of my emotional poise.

When the hurricanes of life, storms of suffering and unplanned circumstances are swirling around you, your inner calm is there for you while your outer life works out the kinks.

You may think none of this applies to you, and maybe it doesn't, but if you are like the rest of us, and we are all pretty much the same, it has its applications.

In the code, the more greens you consume, the sunnier your forecast. If I were to apply the code to emotional poise, it would be the more greens you consume, the more stable your inner life.

When it comes to emotional poise, it's like a muscle, use it or lose it. The next time a person or circumstance aggravates you to overreact, use your emotional poise muscle. Be calm and let them be.

Then drink more greens and be sanguine.

THOUGHT OF THE DAY:

I can't control others but I can control myself.

_____

_____

_____

_____

_____

_____

_____

_____

_____

_____

Bright Morning Green Smoothie

Makes 3 cups or 24 ounces

1 c Water

1 **Cucumber,** cut into 4 pieces – *240g or 8 oz*

1 small **Lemon,** peeled, pith okay, remove seeds – *60g or 2 oz*

3 **Medjool Dates,** pitted – *55g or 2 oz*

2 c **Spinach,** fresh, tightly packed – *100g or 3 ½ oz*

Add the ingredients to your blender in the order listed, blend smooth, approximately 45 seconds. Pour into your favorite glass and savor.

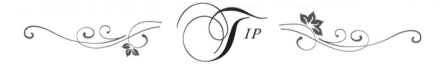

Tip

Beauty Water, as explained on page 240, is also an excellent alternative greens drink for those concerned with sugar and carbohydrate intake.

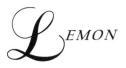

LEMON

Do you want to feel as bright and sunny as a fresh, citrusy lemon? Then make my Bright Morning Green Smoothie and you will.

The 2 cups of spinach in this recipe has 2 grams of protein for your body's building pleasure. The white pith on the lemon helps to nourish the tiny blood vessels in our extremities and assist circulation in our fingertips and toes.

This green smoothie smells bright and sunny, just like the lemon. But it's not a lot of lemon, it's just enough to get you excited and want to drink it. It's tangy but sweet.

Mmm... top of the bright morning to you.

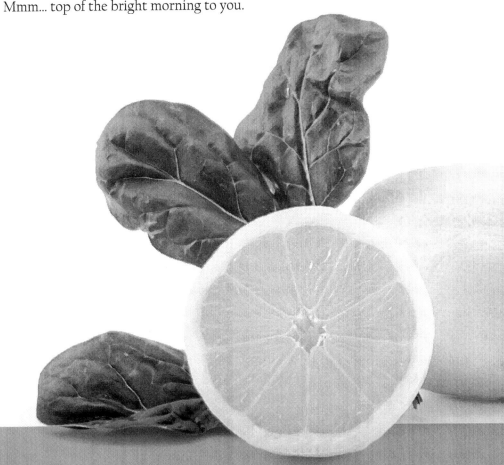

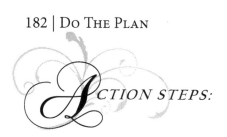

*A*CTION STEPS:

1. Recite today's affirmation aloud three times:

I am practicing emotional poise.

I am practicing emotional poise.

I am practicing emotional poise.

2. Describe a situation in which you delayed overreacting and how the delay improved the outcome.

My Lumen

Check the box that best describes your lumen now:

Daily Greens Consumed		Lumen Forecast	
	Prepare for Planetary Travel		☐
	Sunny Inside and Out		☐
	Partially Sunny		☐
	Cloudy		☐
	Darkness		☐

~400g | ~200g | ~100g | ~50g

On to week four,

here we go...

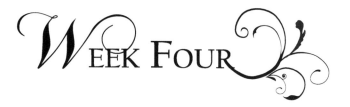

Week Four

"Find the courage to finish."

−Jane

You're in the home stretch of **Green Smoothie Habit**. Enjoy this week's action steps and remember that the greens speak.

They are saying, "Sit up and pay attention. We are nourishing your lumen, which fuels the bright, shining light that is you."

What you are experiencing in **Green Smoothie Habit** is what it's like to create a positive habit from the ground up. You are doing the work and submerging yourself in the process of obtaining and consuming fresh greens. You are including fresh greens in your shopping list. You are putting fresh greens in the forefront of your consciousness and choosing to make it happen.

You are doing the work and you will be rewarded physically, emotionally, mentally and cheerfully by the greens, which have so much to offer us.

Keep going. Don't quit now.

WELCOME TO WEEK 4!

You may be in the last week of **Green Smoothie Habit** but you are in the first days of your new health and wellbeing.

How are you feeling? If you are even one step ahead of where you were when you started, you are succeeding.

Progress is not a straight line. It's a back and forth, twisting, turning, rocket to stardom, nosediving, sometimes random spiral. But, if you just keep moving and making progress, no matter how small or inconsequential you may think it to be, you are moving forward whether you know it or not.

Congratulations on being an action taker. You have mastered the most difficult part. Prepare to finish and enjoy your sense of accomplishment.

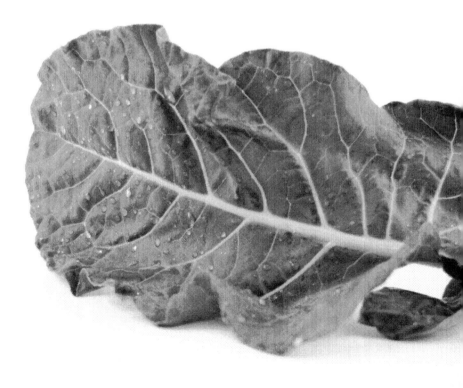

MENU & SHOPPING LIST

DAY 22:	Cilantro Salsa Green Smoothie
DAY 23:	Vital Parsley Green Smoothie
DAY 24:	Lift Off Green Smoothie
DAY 25:	Amazing Kale Green Smoothie
DAY 26:	Honeydew Mint Green Smoothie
DAY 27:	Apple Pie Green Smoothie
DAY 28:	Ginger Salad Green Smoothie

GREENS & VEGGIES

Jalapeño Pepper, 1 (D22)

Cilantro, handful (D22)

Parsley, 1 bunch (D23)

Romaine Lettuce, 3 leaves (D24)

Kale, Red/Russian, 2 leaves (D25)

Ginger, 2 t *fresh* (D25 & 28)

Mint, 1 c *fresh* (D26)

Red Leaf Lettuce, 3 leaves (D27)

Mixed Baby Greens, 1 c (D28)

PANTRY

Sea Salt, ¼ t (D22)

Flax Seed, 1 T *ground* (D27)

FRUIT

Tomatoes, 2 (D22)

Cucumber, 1 (D22)

Limes, 2 (D22, 24, 28)

Red Grapes, 4 c (D23 & 25)

Pineapple, 1 c (D23)

Cantaloupe, 3 c (D24)

Lemon Juice, 1 T (D25)

Honeydew Melon, 5 c (D26 & 28)

Apples, Red Delicious, 3 c (D27)

(D22 = Day 22 etc.) Use this key to help if you shop more than once a week.

Day Twenty-Two

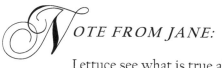

OTE FROM JANE:

Lettuce see what is true about your greens consumption. That's what we're going for here, what is true for you.

This isn't a competition to see who can consume more greens. This is an action guide. To take action, not to be perfect, that is the purpose of **Green Smoothie Habit**.

How do you feel? What is it like to physically shop for greens, inspect them for freshness, place the fresh greens in your cart, purchase them, bring them home, store them, wash them, blend them and sip and savor them?

It's quite a commitment, isn't it?

Isn't it wonderful to not have to think about taking food items away from yourself? To not have to fill your mind space with what you can't eat? This is the spirit of food abundance instead of the spirit of food poverty that dieting creates.

I love the calmness and fun that food abundance offers. It opens my life up. It doesn't reduce and close it down and that's what I want for you.

*T*HOUGHT OF THE DAY:

*The important thing
is to complete*
Green Smoothie Habit.

Cilantro Salsa Green Smoothie

Makes 2 cups or 16 ounces

2 medium Tomatoes – *250g or 9 oz*

1 Cucumber, cut into 4 pieces – *210g or 7 ½ oz*

½" Jalapeño Pepper, remove seeds – *7g or ¼ oz*

1 T Lime Juice, fresh

1 large handful Cilantro – *35g or 1 ¼ oz*

¼ t Sea Salt *optional*

Add the ingredients to your blender in the order listed, blend smooth, approximately 45 seconds. Pour into your favorite glass and savor.

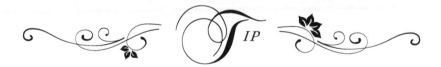

Tip

Drink cilantro, known as the happy herb. It assists in the removal of heavy metals from the body, aiding physical and mental detoxification and clarity.

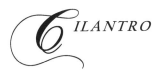

CILANTRO

My Cilantro Salsa Green Smoothie is spiced up with jalapeño pepper, but not too much, just enough for a cleansing kick.

Capsaicin, the chemical that makes chili peppers hot, is a mucous clearing, congestion combatting, sinus infection fighting anti–bacterial agent.

Mixed with Cilantro, a heavy metal removing, anti-fungal herb, we have a powerful, aromatic, delicious and lively libation served up in a margarita glass and it's calling your name. ¡Vamanos!

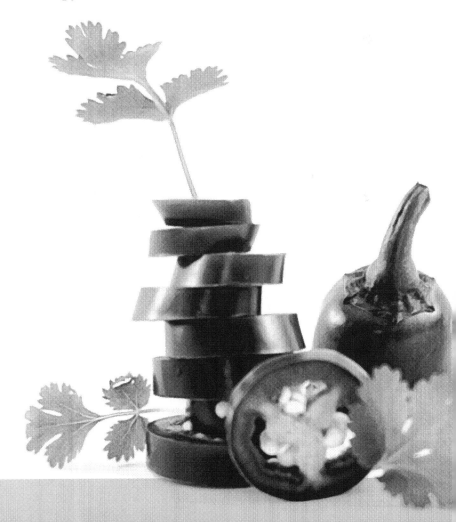

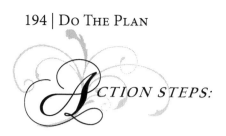

ACTION STEPS:

1. Recite today's affirmation aloud three times:

I am finishing what I start.

I am finishing what I start.

I am finishing what I start.

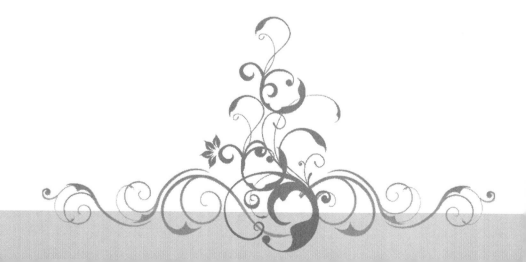

2. List three activities to keep you busy so food isn't all you think about.

Day Twenty-Three

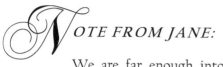

OTE FROM JANE:

We are far enough into **Green Smoothie Habit** to have a discussion about the relationship between fear and energy. Many of us have developed the habit of squelching our energy because we don't know what to do with it.

We have confused energy with fear to the point of being afraid of our energy. Many times, fear is actually your energy trying to get through to you, to see if you are still alive in there. We are trained to think that all energy is physical.

I believe our energy has its own intelligence specific to each of us. That intelligence includes our intuition and our lumen, nourished by our greens consumption.

You are just scratching the surface in these 28 days. I am at seven years of drinking my greens and my energy is an exciting roller coaster, taking me up and down, over and around. The pay off is ongoing. I see no reason why it won't pay off for you. Your energy is a circle of trust between you and your choice to nourish your lumen with the chlorophyll and oxygen of life.

Then a funny thing happens. Energy creates action which crowds out fear. You begin to make the daily, small choices that you used to avoid. You begin to win and fear begins to lose.

You are choosing to treat yourself like the miracle you are. There will never be another you. Never will another human being be you. Never.

THOUGHT OF THE DAY:

It's not about changing who you are...

...it's about letting the greens enhance you.

VITAL PARSLEY GREEN SMOOTHIE

MAKES 4 CUPS OR 32 OUNCES

1 c Water

2 c Red Grapes

1 c Pineapple, fresh or frozen

1 bunch Parsley – *100g or 3 ½ oz*

1 c Ice

Add the ingredients to your blender in the order listed, blend smooth, approximately 45 seconds. Pour into your favorite glass and savor.

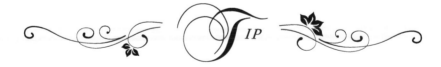

TIP

Why not combine blending and juicing? My Beauty Water Formula on page 241 does just that, giving you the benefits of a green smoothie with the texture of fresh juice.

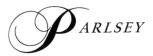

PARLSEY

Simple, refreshing and sweet. This delectable concoction will leave you feeling vital and valuable, and that's a good a thing. It's easy and potent, counteracting toxins eaten and absorbed.

Parsley is anti-bacterial and anti-fungal, sweetening our breath and our thoughts alike.

I enjoy the simplicity, the sweetness and the refreshing ahh... of this smoothie. I hope you do, too.

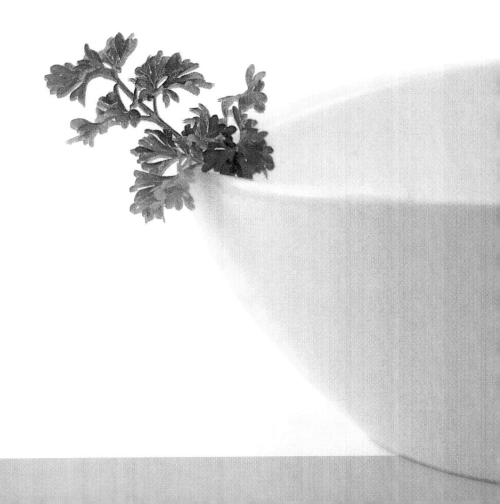

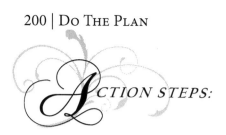

ACTION STEPS:

1. Recite today's affirmation aloud three times:

I am winning, fear is losing.

I am winning, fear is losing.

I am winning, fear is losing.

2. List one positive action you can take that represents fear losing and you winning.

Day Twenty-Four

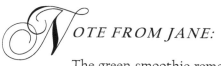

OTE FROM JANE:

The green smoothie remodel you are conducting on yourself is an act of love. Inside and out you will be more beautiful and more vibrant than ever, all because you are taking action and drinking your greens.

Congratulations of the highest order are in order for you. If we were in Camelot you would be knighted by King Arthur. I touch your shoulders with the tip of my sword.

Now, I want to flip you upside down and bring up the other side of taking action. The flip side of the taking action coin are those actions you do not take. The acts not taken because you have replaced acts of self harm with acts of self love.

Perhaps you replaced soda pop with water, sitting with walking, frustration with patience, dreaming with doing. These are expressions of love. You choose a positive action because you love and respect yourself.

Both sides of the taking action coin are nourished by drinking your greens. It is so, no matter my inadequate explanations for the miracle of the greens.

THOUGHT OF THE DAY:

Following your dream is fine...

...but you've got to be a leader to get anything done.

LIFT OFF GREEN SMOOTHIE

MAKES 4 CUPS OR 32 OUNCES

3 c Cantaloupe, ripe

3 leaves Romaine Lettuce – *50g or 2 oz*

2 T Lime Juice, fresh

1 c Ice

Add the ingredients to your blender in the order listed, blend smooth, approximately 45 seconds. Pour into your favorite glass and savor.

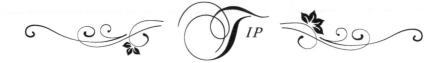

TIP

On page 238, I detail how to tickle the toes of planetary travel and consume two bunches of greens in a day. Think about trying a Two Bunch Bonus Day.

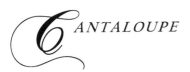

CANTALOUPE

I created this blend because I wanted lift off, like coffee and tea, but without the acidity, so I went for the alkaline greens. Take advantage of Romaine's water, fiber, vitamins, minerals and heart healthy components.

High water content foods like cantaloupe and Romaine lettuce are cleansing, not clogging, healing, not harming. Gives you go–go–go in a good–good way.

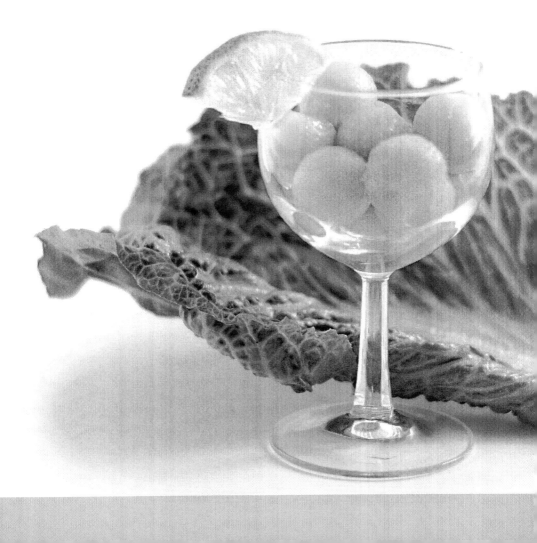

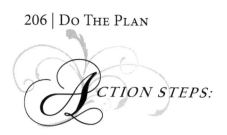

*A*CTION STEPS:

1. Recite today's affirmation aloud three times:

I am able and willing to lead my dream.

I am able and willing to lead my dream.

I am able and willing to lead my dream.

2. Make a note of what actions you did not take because of **Green Smoothie Habit**.

Day Twenty-Five

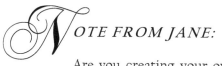

NOTE FROM JANE:

Are you creating your own green smoothies instead of using mine? If so, you're creating a recipe. Write down what's in it, what it tasted like, if you would make it again as is or what you would do to improve it.

The reason I want you to create your own green smoothies is so that, when you finish **Green Smoothie Habit**, you know what to do, how to do it and the habit is established.

If you are doing the action steps, you should be able to fly by now. Staying aloft is something we all struggle with, but that's what GreenSmoothieHabit.com is for, to provide you with a central place of support, community and content.

Green smoothie know how is what holds it all together. When you find yourself alone, when everyone else has quit, when you want to quit, being able to create your own green smoothies will keep you in the game.

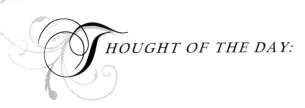

HOUGHT OF THE DAY:

Eat your water.

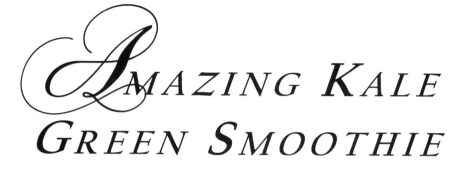

Amazing Kale Green Smoothie

Makes 2 cups or 16 ounces

½ c Water

2 c Red Grapes

2 leaves Red Kale – *25g or 1 oz*

1 T Lemon Juice, fresh

1 t Ginger, fresh – *2g*

Add the ingredients to your blender in the order listed, blend smooth, approximately 45 seconds. Pour into your favorite glass and savor.

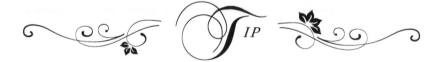

Tip

Keep going. Your Certificate of Achievement awaits you on page 247. Only three days left before you can proudly sign and date it.

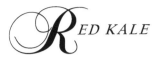

RED KALE

All varieties of kale are rich in chlorophyll, fiber, phytonutrients, anti-oxidants, minerals, vitamins and precious, naturally purified water.

You will be amazed at how the lemon and the ginger enhances the deliciousness of this green smoothie and blends with the grapes for a unique flavor profile.

As I reported on page xvi, we are water. Green smoothies not only help us eat our water but they help us obtain our daily servings of fresh fruits and leafy greens when we might not get them otherwise.

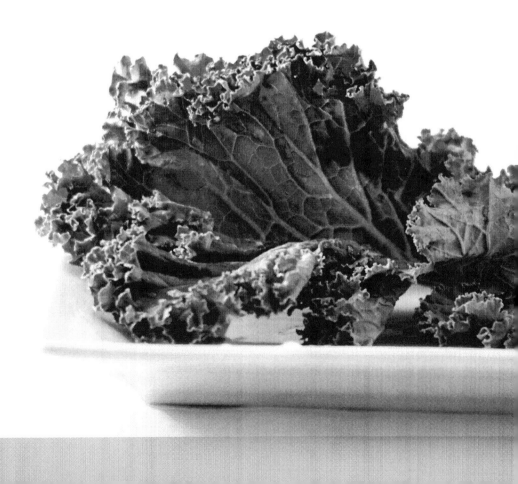

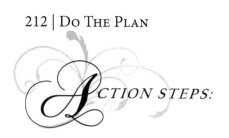

*A*CTION STEPS:

1. Recite today's affirmation aloud three times:

   I am happy and hydrated.

   I am happy and hydrated.

   I am happy and hydrated.

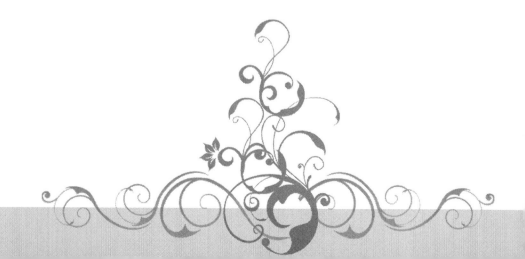

2. How many green smoothies have you created and which one is so delicious you want to share it with others?

DAY TWENTY-SIX

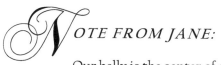

OTE FROM JANE:

Our belly is the center of our body world. Where we go our belly goes. Our belly precedes us into the room and introduces us to others. Our belly advertises us. Our belly holds and processes our nourishment. Our belly is, whether we like it or not, telling others more about us than our faces do.

The reason belly fat is so tough to get rid of is because it is located inside the peritoneal cavity, packed in between internal organs, as opposed to regular fat, which lies just beneath the skin.

If we have excess weight around our middle, we must eliminate it as best we can. In doing so, we remove the possibility of inflammatory secretions. Inflammation is the first step in the disease process.

Our midsections are a suitcase of tension, emotion, and plumbing; a billboard on the highway of our body, warning us, pointing us in the direction we should go, alerting us to construction, detours and crashes.

Our energy intelligence includes our belly and all the organs, muscles and visceral fat it contains. Be patient with yourself and your belly. This is not a race, it's a process in personal improvement.

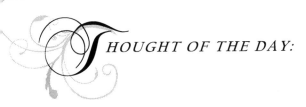

THOUGHT OF THE DAY:

Your belly and you, find out what is true.

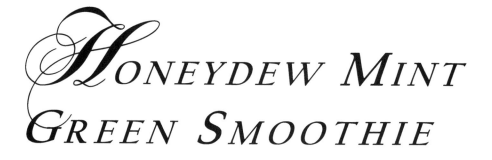

HONEYDEW MINT GREEN SMOOTHIE

MAKES 3 CUPS OR 24 OUNCES

2 c Honeydew Melon, ripe, no seeds
1 c Mint, fresh – *25g or 1 oz*
2 c Ice

Add the ingredients to your blender in the order listed, blend smooth, approximately 45 seconds. Pour into your favorite glass and savor.

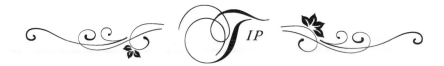

Beautify your table with a bouquet of leafy greens, i.e., rainbow chard and collards. This display will remind you to blend and sip your greens and beautify yourself.

$\mathcal{M}$INT

My frosty Honeydew Mint Green Smoothie will help you through the portal, to the other side where your dreams, motivation and inspiration dwell.

High water content honeydew melon is hydrating and full of minerals and vitamins. Don't overlook it.

And is there anything more refreshing than fresh mint? The aroma is intoxicating and your breath will be as fresh and sweet as this smoothie.

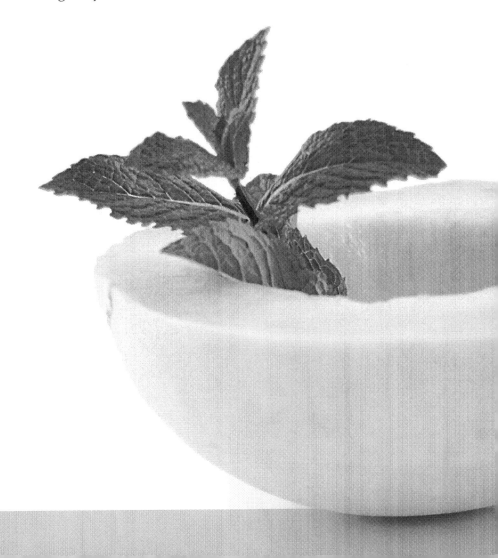

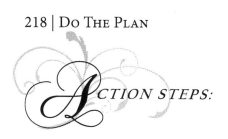

Action steps:

1. Recite today's affirmation aloud three times:

I am thankful for my hard working belly.

I am thankful for my hard working belly.

I am thankful for my hard working belly.

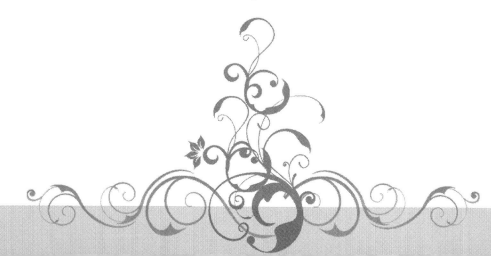

2. Wrap a tape measure around the widest part of your belly and write the number down.

Day Twenty-Seven

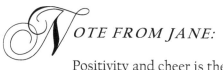

OTE FROM JANE:

Positivity and cheer is the greens drinking outcome for which I am most grateful. It is the aspect that cemented the good habit for me.

If you have been drinking your greens daily, and I hope you have, you will be gifted with good moods and insight, both included in the energy intelligence that comes with the greens.

There are no guarantees that you are going to spend the rest of your life happy just because you drink your greens. Positivity and cheer are better than happiness. Happiness is fleeting, a burst of feeling that usually lasts as long as the conditions that created it.

But positivity and cheer is a foundation skill that carries you through when conditions for happiness do not exist or have gone dormant. Positivity and cheer are brown rice workhorses, while happiness is a few hours of white sugar wonder.

Even when I am not feeling so positive or cheerful, the green smoothie habit carries me through. That's the gift. Being able to carry on is a habit that drinking my greens helped me establish.

When I think of my unalienable right to the pursuit of happiness, the operative word for me is pursuit, not happiness. It's in the daily work of the pursuit that we create our happy outcome.

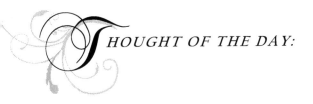

THOUGHT OF THE DAY:

Check the happy box.

Happy ☐

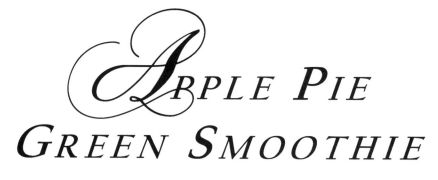

Apple Pie Green Smoothie

Makes 3 cups or 24 ounces

1 c Water

3 c Red Delicious Apples, quartered, remove stems and seeds – *335g or 12 oz*

1 T Flax Seed, ground

⅛ t Cinnamon

3 leaves Red Leaf Lettuce – *100g or 3 ½ oz*

1 c Ice

Add the ingredients to your blender in the order listed, blend smooth, approximately 45 seconds. Pour into your favorite glass and savor.

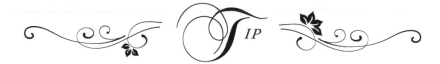

Tip

On page 243 I have compiled a Happy Habit reference list of 32 greens and 37 fruits to ignite your blending imagination and banish boredom.

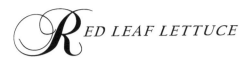ED LEAF LETTUCE

This green smoothie tastes like apple pie and is mmm, mmm, good.

The chlorophyll in the tender red leaf lettuce carries iron and oxygen to our cells and promotes regularity in mind, body and bowel. Flax seed is rich not only in fiber, but the friendly Omega 3 fatty acids that we need.

Choice: Being well.

Result: Well being.

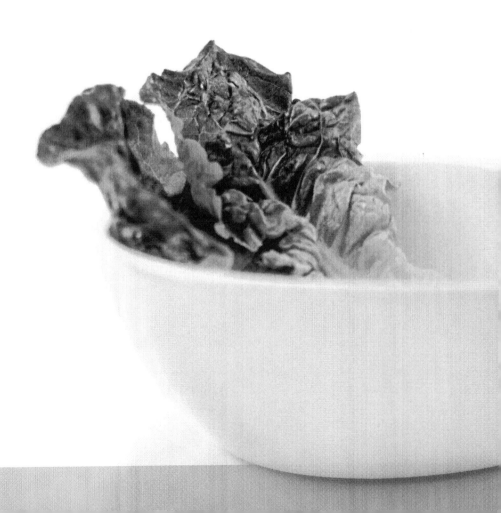

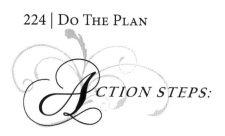

CTION STEPS:

1. Recite today's affirmation aloud three times:

I am in charge of my thoughts.

I am in charge of my thoughts.

I am in charge of my thoughts.

2. Smile.

Day Twenty-Eight

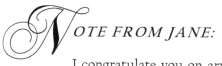

OTE FROM JANE:

I congratulate you on arriving at this day in **Green Smoothie Habit**. Bravo!

When you began, and weekly thereafter, you've rated your lumen.

Your Lumen Forecast is a light meter, not only physical and mental light, but the spiritual light and inner strength required to be proud of who you are and how you live. The greens are foundational, and what they really do is open doors. Will you step through these mystery doors or slam them shut on yourself?

What are you going to do with your new energy? The ideas, thoughts, projects? Will you choose one to complete, step by step?

What are you going to do with the emotional poise that makes it possible for you to carry on and put one foot in front of the other to cross that rickety bridge 500 feet above the raging waters?

Do you go forth into the unknown or stay put? Only you can decide.

THOUGHT OF THE DAY:

How hungry are you?

I don't mean for food...

I mean how motivated are you to continue drinking your greens?

GINGER SALAD GREEN SMOOTHIE

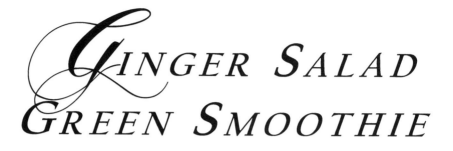

MAKES 2 ½ CUPS OR 20 OUNCES

3 c Honeydew Melon, ripe

1 c Mixed Baby Greens

1 T Lime Juice, fresh

1 t Ginger, fresh – 2g

Add the ingredients to your blender in the order listed, blend smooth, approximately 45 seconds. Pour into your favorite glass and savor.

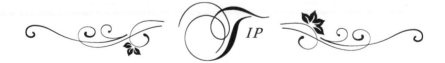

TIP

Do the Special Assignment on page 244.

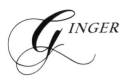

GINGER

Sweet and juicy honeydew melon, a squeeze of lime and a big handful of mixed salad greens blend into a creamy, cooling concoction with the cleansing element of fresh ginger.

Lime brings out the flavor in food and is an alkaline, mineral rich citrus fruit. It may taste tart, but it digests neutral.

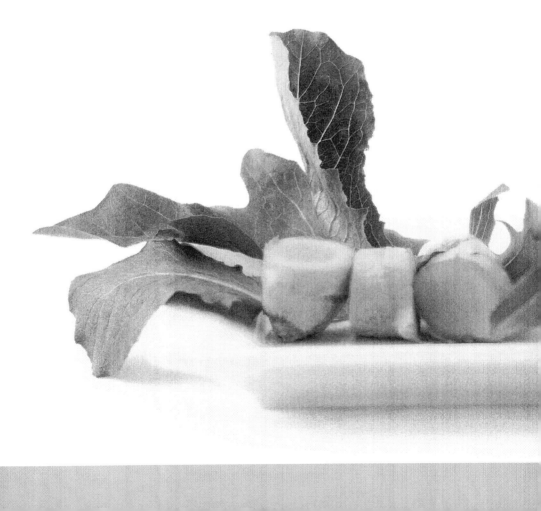

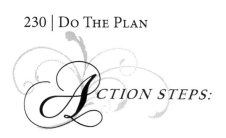

*A*CTION STEPS:

1. Recite today's affirmation aloud three times:

   I am feeding my dreams
   at the cellular level.

   I am feeding my dreams at
   the cellular level.

   I am feeding my dreams at
   the cellular level.

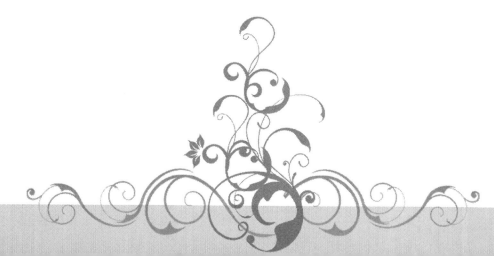

2. List 3 attributes you admire and respect about yourself.

My Lumen

Check the box that best describes your lumen now:

Daily Greens Consumed		Lumen Forecast	
	Prepare for Planetary Travel		☐
	Sunny Inside and Out		☐
	Partially Sunny		☐
	Cloudy		☐
	Darkness		☐

~400g | ~200g | ~100g | ~50g

Turn the page

to cross the finish line...

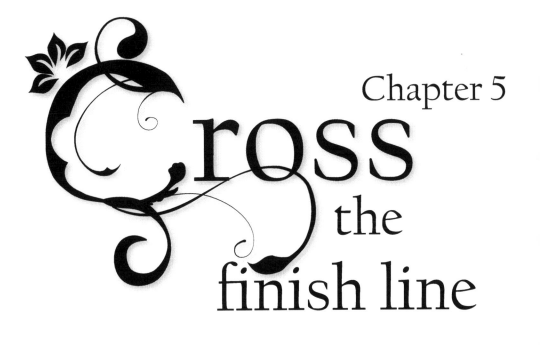

Chapter 5

Cross the finish line

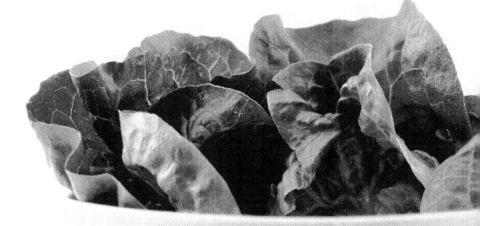

5 | CROSS THE FINISH LINE

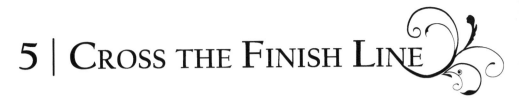

"Congratulations on finishing! You are a pioneer, a leader and a beacon to others."

–Jane

Without you, **Green Smoothie Habit** would have had a hole in it. Your choice to participate means you need and want your lumen and your lumen needs and wants you.

The key is your dream. Is it important, vital and compelling enough to you to take action?

Before you go on to the next page, revisit Chapter 1, page 7 and circle the areas in which you have experienced improvement. Record other improvements you may have experienced, too.

Then revisit Chapter 3, page 30 and reread what you wanted to find on the other side of the green smoothie portal. Does it still resonate? If not, revise it. Either way, don't stop now. Continue your success by adding my three easy methods on the following pages to your green smoothie habit and you are sure to win: Two Bunch Bonus Days, Beauty Water Formula and Happy Habit. Remember to complete the Special Assignment Action Step at the end of this section.

Two Bunch Bonus Days

If you'd like to know what it's like to consume two bunches of greens in a day and tickle the toes of planetary travel as revealed in the code, I have created this one day menu based on what I do when I want to intensify my lumen.

You can eat whatever else you want on a Two Bunch Bonus Day, but I don't have room. It takes me all day to consume the following:

½ gallon Green Smoothie

Made with one bunch of greens using your favorite greens and fruit.
The standard Vitamix container is 64 ounces or ½ gallon.

1 large Salad

Made with one bunch of greens and your favorite salad additions.
Dress with homemade salad dressing, recipes on next page.

I enjoy Two Bunch Bonus Days. Talk about planetary travel... life takes on the heady buzz of wellbeing and time becomes a continuum into which day and night dissolve. You can't help but work on your dream. Two Bunch Bonus Days are my simplest, most joyous and most productive. All is well with the world.

Observe the outcome on your Two Bunch Bonus Days; how you feel, think, react and most importantly, how you replace fear with positive action. That is the measure of results.

SALAD DRESSING RECIPES

The dressings I offer for your salad are so delicious, I couldn't decide which one to use, so here are both of them. They can be used as dips, too.

Add the ingredients to your blender in the order listed and blend smooth.

Peppercorn Ranch Salad Dressing
MAKES 1 ½ CUPS

> 1 c Almond Milk
>
> 1 Avocado
>
> 1 clove Garlic
>
> 8 whole Peppercorns
>
> ½ t Sea Salt
>
> 1 Lemon, juiced
>
> 1 T Nutritional Yeast Flakes, *not Brewer's yeast*

Dancing Dill Salad Dressing
MAKES 1 ½ CUPS

> 1 c Almond Milk
>
> 1 Avocado
>
> 1 clove Garlic
>
> 8 whole Peppercorns
>
> ½ t Sea Salt
>
> 1 Lemon, juiced
>
> 1 handful Dill, fresh

BEAUTY WATERS

There's more than one way to feed your green smoothie habit. Why not include my Beauty Waters? I provide many Beauty Water blends at GreenSmoothieHabit.com.

I created Beauty Water as an alternative greens drink for those concerned with sugar and carbohydrate intake, for those who want a change from thick smoothies and for those who want a craving killing, greens delivering, lumen igniting beverage, not a meal replacement. Water is the base instead of fruit and the amount of greens is reduced.

Beauty Water also solves the juicing versus blending question. It doesn't have to be either/or. Why not combine juicing and blending? Beauty Water does just that. My Beauty Water blends retain the fiber of green smoothies and the texture of juice and can be made in a blender. There's no need to buy an additional appliance such as an expensive juicer.

Sweeteners are optional in Beauty Water. A pitted date, drizzle of honey, or small piece of fruit all work, but are not required. Have some leftover greens? Blend, sip and beautify. Try a squeeze of lemon, lime or orange juice for zing. My simple Beauty Water Formula works every time.

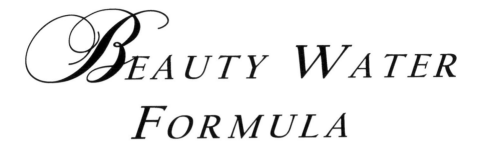

BEAUTY WATER FORMULA

MAKES 6 ½ CUPS

6 c Water

2 leaves or ½ c Greens

Optional Additions:

Ginger Root, Chia Seeds, Dates, Garlic,
Honey, Lemon, Lime, Orange, Blackberries,
Blueberries, Strawberries, Goji Berries,
Green Tea, Aloe, Jalapeño Pepper, Sea Salt,
Cinnamon, Vanilla

HAPPY HABIT

While there are hundreds of delicious and free green smoothie recipes at GreenSmoothieHabit.com, I used only 28 of the simplest blends in this guide to make it as easy as possible for you to get your greens.

Also, for your long term blending convenience I am including a list of greens and fruits to ignite your blending imagination and banish boredom. Mix and match greens and fruit to suit yourself. We all have our favorites, but don't forget to rotate your greens. Fly, green smoothie bird, fly.

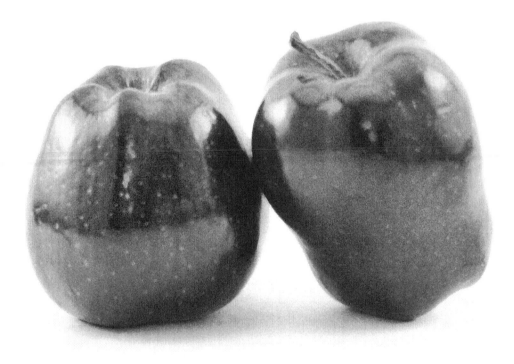

32 GREENS & VEGGIES

Alfalfa Sprouts
Aloe Vera
Arugula
Basil
Beet Greens
Bok Choy
Carrot Greens
Celery
Chard
Cilantro
Collard Greens

Dandelion
Dill
Grapeleaves
Kale
Lambsquarters
Lettuce, Butterhead
Lettuce, Endive
Lettuce, Green Leaf
Lettuce, Iceberg
Lettuce, Red Leaf
Lettuce, Romaine

Mint
Mustard Greens
Oregano
Parsley
Purslane
Rosemary
Sorrel
Spinach
Turnip Greens
Watercress

37 FRUITS

Apple
Apricot
Asian Pear
Avocado
Banana
Bell Pepper, yellow, red, orange
Blackberry
Blueberry
Cantaloupe
Cherry
Coconut Meat and Water

Cranberry
Cucumber
Date
Fig
Grape
Grapefruit
Kiwi
Lemon
Lime
Mango
Melon
Nectarine
Orange

Papaya
Peach
Pear
Persimmon
Pineapple
Plum
Pomegranate
Prune
Raspberry
Starfruit
Strawberry
Tangerine
Tomato

SPECIAL ASSIGNMENT

I'm going to ask you to take a big risk in the special assignment below. Nobody can read what you will write unless you show it to them. I am rooting for you.

Reveal your dream. You know the one. The dream you dare not voice for fear of ridicule and weakness, yet you cannot stop the longing. Use the "W" words as a guide and reveal your dream:

Who:

What:

When:

Where:

Why:

How:

SO LONG, NOT GOODBYE

You have an inner light that is a physical place in your body, like a city on a map. It has a name, lumen, and is a destination inside your blood vessels and intestines that can be nourished with your food, drink and thoughts.

I believe our lumen has markers, like our blood, fingerprints and irises, to identify that light as our own, so we can find each other in eternity.

Drink your greens, nourish your light and you will soon revel in your Lumen Forecast. It is what **Green Smoothie Habit** shows and my experience proves. You've never been more beautiful.

Meet me at...

GreenSmoothieHabit.com/myHabit

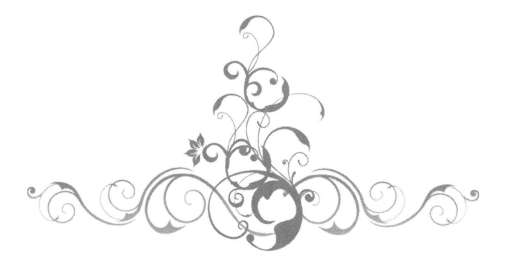

Certificate of Achievement

is hereby congratulated on completing

Green Smoothie Habit

Drink Your Greens To Achieve Your Dreams 28 Day Success Guide

on _____ , 20 _____

Jane Haddad

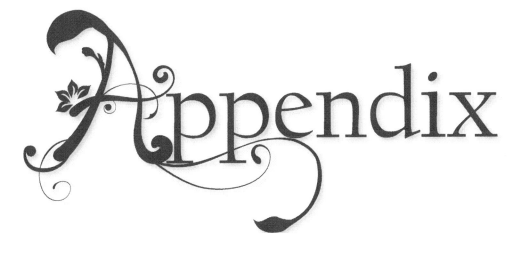

Appendix

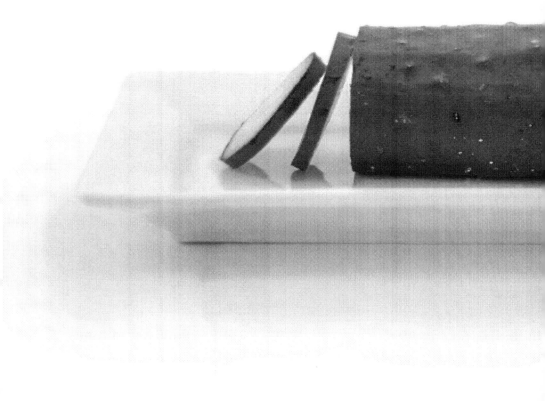

APPENDIX

GREEN SMOOTHIE MAKING TIPS

1. Wash greens and fruit before using.

2. Peel and remove seeds and pits from fruit.

3. Remove tough stems on kale, chard, collards, etc.

4. Keep tender stems on parsley, cilantro, lettuces, etc.

5. Rotate your greens. Today kale, tomorrow chard, etc. This is the most important tip I can give you. Greens contain alkaloids and the human body has no trouble eliminating them, but you don't want to build up a large store of any one of them. 7 different greens in 7 days is ideal.

6. If in doubt on proportions, let ⅔ fruit, ⅓ greens be your guide.

7. Too green? Add fruit.

8. Too sweet? Add greens.

9. Grapes with seeds are fine in a high speed blender.

10. To freeze bananas, place ripe (make sure the peels have the brown sugar spots), peeled bananas into a freezer bag and they will keep for approximately two weeks.

11. Load ingredients into your blender as follows: liquids, fruit, greens, ice.

12. Best made in a high speed blender but not required. If you don't have a high speed blender, work with what you have. You may have to cut the recipe in half or thirds or add more water or leave out the ice to get it to blend. It may not be as smooth as you like, but that's okay. Do something, start somewhere.

AFFIRMATIONS

Day 1: I am alive and feeling good.

Day 2: I am kind to me, too.

Day 3: I am strong.

Day 4: I am relaxed and safe.

Day 5: I am taking action and it feels good.

Day 6: I am worth taking care of.

Day 7: I am confident and capable.

Day 8: I am eating well.

Day 9: I am respecting my colon.

Day 10: I am enjoying leafy greens.

Day 11: I am aware change is difficult, but I can do it.

Day 12: I am valuable.

Day 13: I am drinking my greens.

Day 14: I am free to choose my attitude.

Day 15: I am improving myself.

Day 16: I am glad I am nourishing my lumen.

Day 17: I am not afraid.

Day 18: I am responsible for myself and I like it.

Day 19: I am creative.

Day 20: I am completing today's action steps.

Day 21: I am practicing emotional poise.

Day 22: I am finishing what I start.

Day 23: I am winning, fear is losing.

Day 24: I am able and willing to lead my dream.

Day 25: I am happy and hydrated.

Day 26: I am thankful for my hard working belly.

Day 27: I am in charge of my thoughts.

Day 28: I am feeding my dreams at the cellular level.

MEASUREMENT GUIDE & CONVERSIONS

Teaspoons	Tablespoons	Cups	Quantity
¼ t			
½ t			
1 t			⅙ oz
3 t	1 T		½ oz
	2 T		1 oz
	8 T	½ c	4 oz
	16 T	1 c	8 oz

GREEN SMOOTHIE HABIT
28 DAY SUCCESS GUIDE RECIPES

Week 1 Recipes: Days 1 – 7

DAY 1: Who Knew?

1 Tomato
1 Cucumber, cut into 4 pieces
½ head Iceberg Lettuce
¼ t Sea Salt *optional*

DAY 2: Feel Better

4 c Apple Juice, fresh
2–3 leaves Lacinato/Dinosaur
    Kale – *any variety kale*
½ t Cinnamon
2 T Lemon Juice, fresh

DAY 3: Beautiful Skin

1 Ruby Red Grapefruit, remove
    peel, pith, skin and seeds
1 Cucumber, cut into 4 pieces
¾ bunch Parsley, fresh
    substitute any variety parsley
1 handful Mint, fresh

DAY 4: Thirst Quencher

1 c Water
½ c Orange Juice, fresh
1 ½ c Pineapple, cubed, fresh or
    frozen
4–6 leaves Romaine Lettuce
1 Banana, ripe, fresh or frozen

DAY 5: Carrot Top

1 c Water
5 c Red Delicious Apples,
    cubed (about 3 apples)
1 handful Carrot Tops/Greens
1 handful Mint, fresh
½ c Ice

DAY 6: Anti–Oxidant

1 c Water
3 c Blueberries, fresh or frozen
2–3 leaves Collard Greens,
    stems removed
4 Bananas, ripe, fresh or frozen
2 c Ice *optional*

DAY 7: Cherry Chard

1 ½ c Water
2 c Cherries, pitted, fresh or
    frozen
2–3 leaves Chard, cut off
    bottom stems
2 c Ice

Week 2 Recipes: Days 8–14

DAY 8: **Easy Spinach**

> 4 c Green Grapes, sweet
> ½ bunch Spinach
> 2 c Ice

DAY 9: **Well Being**

> 4 c Red Grapes, sweet
> 1 bunch Beet Greens
> 1 T Flax Seed, ground
> 2 c Ice

DAY 10: **Bok Choy Cheer**

> 3 c Tangerine Juice, fresh
>   squeezed
> 2–3 Bok Choy leaves or 1
>   bunch Baby Bok Choy
> 2–3 sprigs Mint, fresh

DAY 11: **Watercress Zing**

> 1 c Water
> 1 Cucumber, cut into 4 pieces
> 1 c Watercress or Upland
>   Cress
> 1 T Lemon Juice, fresh
> ½ t Sea Salt *optional*

DAY 12: **Dandelion Eyes**

> 4 Oranges, sweet & juicy,
>   peeled, remove seeds
> 4 leaves Dandelion
> 1 c Ice

DAY 13: **Good Mood**

> 2 c Water
> 1 Cucumber, cut into 4 pieces
> ¼ c Dill, fresh, lightly packed
> 2 Medjool Dates, pitted

DAY 14: **Papaya Basil**

> 3 c ripe Papaya, fresh
> ¼ c Basil, fresh
> 1 t Lime Juice, fresh
> 1 c Ice

Week 3 Recipes: Days 15–21

DAY 15: **Endless Endive**

3 c Watermelon, remove rind and seeds
1 handful Curly Endive, also known as Frisée
1 t Lemon Juice, fresh

DAY 16: **Kale Beauty**

2 c Red Grapes
2 c Mango, fresh or frozen
3 leaves Curly Kale
1 c Ice

DAY 17: **Quiet Time**

1 c Water
2 c Nectarines, ripe
2 leaves Butter Head/Bibb Lettuce

DAY 18: **Pear Party**

1 c Water
2 c Pears, ripe
1 c Mixed Baby Greens

DAY 19: **Electrolyte**

4 Roma/Plum Tomatoes
2 stalks Celery, save the leafy tips for garnish
1 T Lime Juice, fresh
¼ t Sea Salt *optional*
Pinch Black Pepper, fresh ground

DAY 20: **Potassium Power**

1 c Water
2 Bananas, ripe, fresh or frozen
2 leaves Green Leaf Lettuce
1 c Ice

DAY 21: **Bright Morning**

1 c Water
1 Cucumber, cut into 4 pieces
1 small Lemon, peeled, pith okay, remove seeds
3 Medjool Dates, pitted
2 c Spinach, fresh, tightly packed

Week 4 Recipes: Days 22–28

DAY 22: Cilantro Salsa

2 medium Tomatoes
1 Cucumber, cut into 4 pieces
½" Jalapeño Pepper, remove
   seeds
1 T Lime Juice, fresh
1 large handful Cilantro
¼ t Sea Salt *optional*

DAY 23: Vital Parsley

1 c Water
2 c Red Grapes
1 c Pineapple, fresh or frozen
1 bunch Parsley
1 c Ice

DAY 24: Lift Off

3 c Cantaloupe, ripe
3 leaves Romaine Lettuce
2 T Lime Juice, fresh
1 c Ice

DAY 25: Amazing Kale

½ c Water
2 c Red Grapes
2 leaves Red Kale
1 T Lemon Juice, fresh
1 t Ginger, fresh

DAY 26: Honeydew Mint

2 c Honeydew Melon, ripe ,no
   seeds
1 c Mint, fresh
2 c Ice

DAY 27: Apple Pie

1 c Water
3 c Red Delicious Apples,
   quartered, remove stems and
   seeds
1 T Flax Seed, ground
⅛ t Cinnamon
3 leaves Red Leaf Lettuce
1 c Ice

DAY 28: Ginger Salad

3 c Honeydew Melon, ripe
1 c Mixed Baby Greens
1 T Lime Juice, fresh
1 t Ginger, fresh

Bonus Day Dressing: Recipes & Shopping List

Recipes

DRESSING 1: **Peppercorn Ranch**

1 c Almond Milk
1 Avocado
1 clove Garlic
8 whole Peppercorns
½ t Sea Salt
1 Lemon, juiced
1 T Nutritional Yeast Flakes,
    not Brewer's yeast

DRESSING 2: **Dancing Dill**

1 c Almond Milk
1 Avocado
1 clove Garlic
8 whole Peppercorns
½ t Sea Salt
1 Lemon, juiced
1 handful Dill, fresh

Shopping List

PRODUCE

Avocado, 1
Garlic, 1 clove
Lemon, 1
Dill, 1 handful *fresh* (DD)

PANTRY

Almond Milk, 1 c
Peppercorns, 8 whole
Sea Salt, ½ t
Nutritional Yeast Flakes, 1 T,
    not Brewer's yeast (PR)

(PR = Peppercorn Ranch, DD = Dancing Dill) Use this key to help you distinguish salad dressings when shopping.

Shopping Lists

Week 1 Shopping List: Days 1-7

GREENS & VEGGIES

Iceburg Lettuce, ½ head (D1)

Lacinato/Dinosaur Kale, 2 – 3 leaves (D2)

Parsley, ¾ bunch *any variety* (D3)

Mint, 2 handfuls *fresh* (D3 & 5)

Romaine Lettuce, 4–6 leaves(D4)

Carrot Top/Greens, handful(D5)

Collard Greens, 2 – 3 leaves (D6)

Chard, 2 – 3 leaves (D7)

PANTRY

Sea Salt, ¼ t (D1)

Cinnamon, ½ t (D2)

FRUIT

Tomato, 1 (D1)

Cucumbers, 2 (D1 & 3)

Apple Juice, 4 c *fresh* (D2)

Lemon Juice, 2 T *fresh* (D2)

Grapefruit, 1 (D3)

Orange Juice, ½ c *fresh* (D4)

Pineapple, 1 ½ c cubed *fresh or frozen* (D4)

Bananas, 5 *ripe* (D4 & 6)

Red Delicious Apples, 5 c chopped, *approx. 3 apples* (D5)

Blueberries, 3 c *fresh or frozen* (D6)

Cherries, 2 c pitted, *fresh or frozen* (D7)

Week 2 Shopping List: Days 8-14

GREENS & VEGGIES

Spinach, ½ bunch (D8)

Beet Greens, 1 bunch (D9)

Bok Choy, 2 leaves or 1 bunch Baby Bok Choy (D10)

Mint, 3 sprigs *fresh* (D10)

Watercress, 1 c (D11)

Dandelion, 4 leaves (D12)

Dill, ¼ c *fresh* (D13)

Basil, ¼ c *fresh* (D14)

PANTRY

Flax Seed, 1 T *ground* (D9)

Sea Salt, ½ t (*optional*) (D11)

FRUIT

Green Grapes, 4 c (D8)

Red Grapes, 4 c (D9)

Tangerine Juice, 3 c (D10)

Cucumber, 2 (D11, D13)

Lemon Juice, 1 T *fresh* (D11)

Oranges, 4 (D12)

Medjool Dates, 2 (D13)

Papaya, 3 c (D14)

Lime Juice, 1 t *fresh* (D14)

Week 3 Shopping List: Days 15–21

GREENS & VEGGIES

Curly Endive, handful (D15)

Curly Kale, 3 leaves (D16)

Butter Head/Bibb Lettuce, 2 leaves (D17)

Mixed Baby Greens, 1 c (D18)

Celery, 2 stalks with leafy tips (D19)

Green Leaf Lettuce, 2 leaves (D20)

Spinach, 2 c (D21)

PANTRY

Sea Salt, ¼ t *optional*,(D19)

Black Pepper, pinch *ground* (D19)

FRUIT

Watermelon, 3 c (D15)

Lemon Juice, 1 t *fresh* (D15)

Grapes, Red 2 c (D16)

Mango, 2 c *fresh or frozen* (D16)

Nectarines, 2 c (D17)

Pears, 2 c (D18)

Tomatoes, Roma, 4 (D19)

Lime Juice, 1 T *fresh* (D19)

Bananas, 2 (D20)

Cucumber, 1 (D21)

Lemon, 1 (D21)

Medjool Dates, 3 (D21)

Week 4 Shopping List: Days 22–28

GREENS & VEGGIES

Jalapeño Pepper, 1 (D22)

Cilantro, handful (D22)

Parsley, 1 bunch (D23)

Romaine Lettuce, 3 leaves (D24)

Kale, Red, 2 leaves (D25)

Ginger, 2 t *fresh* (D25 & 28)

Mint, 1 c *fresh* (D26)

Red Leaf Lettuce, 3 leaves (D27)

Mixed Baby Greens, 1 c(D28)

PANTRY

Sea Salt, ¼ t (D22)

Flax Seed, 1 T *ground* (D27)

FRUIT

Tomatoes, 2 (D22)

Cucumber, 1 (D22)

Limes, 2 (D22, 24, 28)

Red Grapes, 4 c (D23, 25)

Pineapple, 1 c (D23)

Cantaloupe, 3 c (D24)

Lemon Juice, 1 T (D25)

Honeydew Melon, 5 c (D26, 28)

Apples, Red Delicious, 3 c (D27)

VITAMIX BLENDER
INFORMATION

My Vitamix high speed blender is the best investment I have made in my health and wellbeing. My life has changed in many positive ways from the thousands of green smoothies I have made in my Vitamix, on camera and off.

I have arranged 3 easy ways for you to purchase this wonderful investment in your health.

To purchase online, over the phone or to arrange a 3-pay plan, please visit this page on my website for up to date details:

GreenSmoothieHabit.com/vitamix

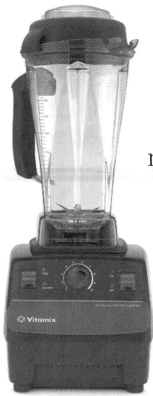

The Vitamix
makes the perfect
green smoothie!

Website Information

Visit GreenSmoothieHabit.com for products, recipes, videos, community and testimonials:

www.GreenSmoothieHabit.com

Bibliography

Boutenko, Victoria. *Green for Life.* [Ashland, OR]: Raw Family Pub., 2005. 80. Print.

"Nutrient Data Laboratory Home Page." *USDA National Nutrient Database for Standard Reference, Release 25.* U.S. Department of Agriculture, Agricultural Research Service, 2012. Web. 25 Apr. 2013. ‹http://www.ars.usda.gov/ba/bhnrc/ndl›

GLYCEMIC INDEX DATA

The Glycemic Index refers to the effect that carbohydrate foods have on blood sugar levels. The number is a comparison with a reference food, usually white bread (70) or glucose (100). Foods with a high number release glucose quickly and cause a rapid rise in blood sugar. Foods with a low number release glucose slowly into the blood.

Fruits Used in Green Smoothie Habit
Glycemic Index Averages Per 100g

Low 0–50   Medium 51–70   High 71–100

Apple	38
Apple Juice, Fresh Squeezed	40
Bananas	52
Blueberries	40
Cantaloupe	65
Cherries	22
Cucumber	32
Dates, Medjool	103
Grapefruit	25
Grapes, Green	46
Grapes, Red	46
Honeydew Melon	65
Mango	56
Nectarine	42
Orange	42
Orange Juice, Fresh Squeezed	50
Papaya	59
Peach	42
Pear	38
Pineapple	59
Tangerine Juice	50
Tomatoes	38
Watermelon	72

GREENS NUTRITIONAL DATA

Greens Used in Green Smoothie Habit

Nutrient Values per 100g Edible Portion

Green	Proximates		Vitamins		Minerals		Amino Acids	
Basil	Water	92.06 g	Vitamin A	5275 IU	Calcium	177 mg	Histidine	51 mg
	Protein	3.15 g	Vitamin B6	0.155 mg	Iron	3.17 mg	Isoleucine	104 mg
	Calories	23	Vitamin C	18.0 mg	Magnesium	64 mg	Leucine	191 mg
			Vitamin E	0.80 mg	Phosphorus	56 mg	Lysine	110 mg
			Vitamin K	414.8 µg	Potassium	295 mg	Methionine	36 mg
			Thiamin	0.034 mg	Sodium	4 mg	Phenylalaline	58 mg
			Riboflavin	0.076 mg	Zinc	0.81 mg	Threonine	130 mg
			Niacin	0.902 mg	Copper	0.385 mg	Tryptophan	39 mg
			Vitamin B5	0.209 mg	Manganese	1.148 mg	Valine	127 mg
			Folate	68 µg	Selenium	0.3 µg		
Beet Greens	Water	91.02 g	Vitamin A	6326 IU	Calcium	117 mg	Histidine	34 mg
	Protein	2.20 g	Vitamin B6	0.106 mg	Iron	2.57 mg	Isoleucine	46 mg
	Calories	22	Vitamin C	30.0 mg	Magnesium	70 mg	Leucine	98 mg
			Vitamin E	1.50 mg	Phosphorus	41 mg	Lysine	64 mg
			Vitamin K	400 µg	Potassium	762 mg	Methionine	18 mg
			Thiamin	0.100 mg	Sodium	226 mg	Phenylalaline	58 mg
			Riboflavin	0.220 mg	Zinc	0.38 mg	Threonine	65 mg
			Niacin	0.400 mg	Copper	0.191 mg	Tryptophan	35 mg
			Vitamin B5	0.250 mg	Manganese	0.391 mg	Valine	65 mg
			Folate	15 µg	Selenium	0.9 µg		
Bok Choy	Water	95.3 g	Vitamin A	4468 IU	Calcium	105 mg	Tryptophan	15 mg
	Protein	1.5 g	Alpha Carotene	1.0 µg	Iron	0.8 mg	Threonine	49 mg
	Calories	13	Beta Carotene	2681 µg	Magnesium	19.0 mg	Isoleucine	85 mg
			Lycopene	0.0 µg	Phosphorus	37.0 mg	Leucine	88 mg
			Vitamin C	45.0 mg	Potassium	252 mg	Lysine	89 mg
			Vitamin E	0.1 mg	Sodium	65.0 mg	Methionine	9 mg
			Vitamin K	45.5 µg	Zinc	0.2 mg	Cystine	17 mg
			Thiamin	0.0 mg	Copper	0.0 mg	Phenylalanine	44 mg
			Riboflavin	0.1 mg	Manganese	0.2 mg	Tyrosine	29 mg
			Niacin	0.5 mg	Selenium	0.5 µg	Valine	66 mg
			Vitamin B6	0.2 mg			Arginine	84 mg
			Folate	66.0 µg			Histidine	26 mg
			Food Folate	66.0 µg			Alanine	86 mg
			Folic Acid	0.0 µg			Aspartic acid	108 mg
			Dietary Folate	66.0 µg			Glutamic acid	360 mg
			Vitamin B12	0.0 µg			Glycine	43 mg
			Vitamin B5	0.1 mg			Proline	31 mg
			Choline	6.4 mg			Serine	48 mg
			Betaine	0.3 mg				

Green	Proximates		Vitamins		Minerals		Amino Acids	
Carrot Greens	N/A		N/A		N/A		N/A	
Chard	Water	92.66 g	Vitamin A	6116 IU	Calcium	51 mg	Histidine	36 mg
	Protein	1.80 g	Vitamin B6	0.099 mg	Iron	1.80 mg	Isoleucine	147 mg
	Calories	19	Vitamin C	30.0 mg	Magnesium	81 mg	Leucine	130 mg
			Vitamin E	1.89 mg	Phosphorus	46 mg	Lysine	99 mg
			Vitamin K	830.0 µg	Potassium	379 mg	Methionine	19 mg
			Thiamin	0.040 mg	Sodium	213 mg	Phenylalaline	110 mg
			Riboflavin	0.090 mg	Zinc	0.36 mg	Threonine	83 mg
			Niacin	0.400 mg	Copper	0.179 mg	Tryptophan	17 mg
			Vitamin B5	0.172 mg	Manganese	0.366 mg	Valine	110 mg
			Folate	14 µg	Selenium	0.9 µg		
Cilantro	Water	92.21 g	Vitamin A	6748 IU	Calcium	67 mg	N/A	
	Protein	2.13 g	Vitamin B6	0.149 mg	Iron	1.77 mg		
	Calories	23	Vitamin C	27.0 mg	Magnesium	26 mg		
			Vitamin E	2.50 mg	Phosphorus	48 mg		
			Vitamin K	310.0 µg	Potassium	521 mg		
			Thiamin	0.067 mg	Sodium	46 mg		
			Riboflavin	0.162 mg	Zinc	0.50 mg		
			Niacin	1.114 mg	Copper	0.225 mg		
			Vitamin B5	0.570 mg	Manganese	0.426 mg		
			Folate	62 µg	Selenium	0.9 µg		
Collard Greens	Water	90.55 g	Vitamin A	6668 IU	Calcium	145 mg	Histidine	47 mg
	Protein	2.45 g	Vitamin B6	0.165 mg	Iron	0.19 mg	Isoleucine	100 mg
	Calories	30	Vitamin C	35.3 mg	Magnesium	9 mg	Leucine	151 mg
			Vitamin E	2.26 mg	Phosphorus	10 mg	Lysine	117 mg
			Vitamin K	510.8 µg	Potassium	169 mg	Methionine	33 mg
			Thiamin	0.054 mg	Sodium	0 mg	Phenylalaline	87 mg
			Riboflavin	0.130 mg	Zinc	0.13 mg	Threonine	86 mg
			Niacin	0.742 mg	Copper	0.039 mg	Tryptophan	31 mg
			Vitamin B5	0.267 mg	Manganese	0.276 mg	Valine	120 mg
			Folate	166 µg	Selenium	1.3 µg		
Dandelion Greens	Water	85.60 g	Vitamin A	10161 IU	Calcium	187 mg	N/A	
	Protein	2.70 g	Vitamin B6	0.251 mg	Iron	3.10 mg		
	Calories	45	Vitamin C	5.0 mg	Magnesium	36 mg		
			Vitamin E	3.44 mg	Phosphorus	66 mg		
			Vitamin K	778.4 µg	Potassium	397 mg		
			Thiamin	0.190 mg	Sodium	76 mg		
			Riboflavin	0.260 mg	Zinc	0.41 mg		
			Niacin	0.806 mg	Copper	0.171 mg		
			Vitamin B5	0.084 mg	Manganese	0.342 mg		
			Folate	27 µg	Selenium	0.5 µg		

Green	Proximates		Vitamins		Minerals		Amino Acids	
Dill	Water	85.95 g	Vitamin A	7718 IU	Calcium	208 mg	Tryptophan	14 mg
	Protein	3.46 g	Vitamin C	85 mg	Iron	6.59 mg	Threonine	68 mg
	Calories	43	Thiamin	.058 mg	Magnesium	55 mg	Isoleucine	195 mg
			Riboflavin	.296 mg	Phosphorus	66 mg	Leucine	159 mg
			Niacin	1.570 mg	Potassium	738 mg	Lysine	246 mg
			Vitamin B6	.185 mg	Sodium	61 mg	Methionine	11 mg
			Folate	15 µg	Zinc	.91 mg	Cystine	17 mg
							Phenylalanine	65 mg
							Tyrosine	96 mg
							Valine	154 mg
							Arginine	142 mg
							Histidine	71 mg
							Alanine	227 mg
							Aspartic acid	343 mg
							Glutamic acid	290 mg
							Glycine	169 mg
							Proline	248 mg
							Serine	158 mg
Kale, Curly	Water	93.79 g	Vitamin A	15376 IU	Calcium	135 mg	Histidine	69 mg
	Protein	1.25 g	Vitamin B6	0.271 mg	Iron	1.70 mg	Isoleucine	197 mg
	Calories	50	Vitamin C	120.0 mg	Magnesium	34 mg	Leucine	231 mg
			Vitamin E	N/A	Phosphorus	56 mg	Lysine	197 mg
			Vitamin K	817.0 µg	Potassium	447 mg	Methionine	32 mg
			Thiamin	0.110 mg	Sodium	43 mg	Phenylalaline	169 mg
			Riboflavin	0.130 mg	Zinc	0.44 mg	Threonine	147 mg
			Niacin	1.000 mg	Copper	0.290 mg	Tryptophan	40 mg
			Vitamin B5	0.091 mg	Manganese	0.774 mg	Valine	181 mg
			Folate	29 µg	Selenium	0.9 µg		
Lettuce, Butterhead/Bibb	Water	95.63 g	Vitamin A	3312 IU	Calcium	35 mg	Histidine	17 mg
	Protein	1.35 g	Vitamin B6	0.082 mg	Iron	1.24 mg	Isoleucine	39 mg
	Calories	13	Vitamin C	3.7 mg	Magnesium	13 mg	Leucine	71 mg
			Vitamin E	0.18 mg	Phosphorus	33 mg	Lysine	56 mg
			Vitamin K	102.3 µg	Potassium	238 mg	Methionine	14 mg
			Thiamin	0.057 mg	Sodium	5 mg	Phenylalaline	53 mg
			Riboflavin	0.062 mg	Zinc	0.20 mg	Threonine	41 mg
			Niacin	0.357 mg	Copper	0.016 mg	Tryptophan	13 mg
			Vitamin B5	0.150 mg	Manganese	0.179 mg	Valine	54 mg
			Folate	73 µg	Selenium	0.6 µg		
Lettuce, Endive	Water	93.79 g	Vitamin A	2167 IU	Calcium	52 mg	Histidine	23 mg
	Protein	1.25 g	Vitamin B6	0.020 mg	Iron	0.83 mg	Isoleucine	72 mg
	Calories	17	Vitamin C	6.5 mg	Magnesium	15 mg	Leucine	98 mg
			Vitamin E	0.44 mg	Phosphorus	28 mg	Lysine	63 mg

Green	Proximates		Vitamins		Minerals		Amino Acids	
Lettuce, Endive, cont'd.			Vitamin K	231.0 µg	Potassium	314 mg	Methionine	14 mg
			Thiamin	0.080 mg	Sodium	22 mg	Phenylalaline	53 mg
			Riboflavin	0.075 mg	Zinc	0.79 mg	Threonine	50 mg
			Niacin	0.400 mg	Copper	0.099 mg	Tryptophan	5 mg
			Vitamin B5	0.900 mg	Manganese	0.420 mg	Valine	63 mg
			Folate	142 µg	Selenium	0.2 µg		

Green	Proximates		Vitamins		Minerals		Amino Acids	
Lettuce, Green Leaf	Water	95.07 g	Vitamin A	7405 IU	Calcium	36 mg	Histidine	22 mg
	Protein	1.36 g	Vitamin B6	0.090 mg	Iron	0.86 mg	Isoleucine	84 mg
	Calories	15	Vitamin C	18.0 mg	Magnesium	13 mg	Leucine	79 mg
			Vitamin E	0.29 mg	Phosphorus	29 mg	Lysine	84 mg
			Vitamin K	173.6 µg	Potassium	194 mg	Methionine	16 mg
			Thiamin	0.070 mg	Sodium	28 mg	Phenylalaline	55 mg
			Riboflavin	0.080 mg	Zinc	0.18 mg	Threonine	59 mg
			Niacin	0.357 mg	Copper	0.029 mg	Tryptophan	9 mg
			Vitamin B5	0.134 mg	Manganese	0.250 mg	Valine	70 mg
			Folate	38 µg	Selenium	0.6 µg		

Green	Proximates		Vitamins		Minerals		Amino Acids	
Lettuce, Iceberg	Water	95.64 g	Vitamin C	2.8 mg	Calcium	18 mg	Tryptophan	9 mg
	Protein	.90 g	Thiamin	.041 mg	Iron	.41 mg	Threonine	25 mg
	Calories	14	Riboflavin	.025 mg	Magnesium	7 mg	Isoleucine	18 mg
			Niacin	.123 mg	Phosphorus	20 mg	Leucine	25 mg
			Vitamin B6	.042 mg	Potassium	141 mg	Lysine	24 mg
			Folate	29 µg	Sodium	10 mg	Methionine	5 mg
			Vitamin A	25 µg	Zinc	.15 mg	Cystine	5 mg
			Vitamin E	.18 mg			Phenylalanine	23 mg
			Vitamin K	24.1 µg			Tyrosine	7 mg
							Valine	24 mg
							Arginine	15 mg
							Histidine	9 mg
							Alanine	25 mg
							Aspartic acid	125 mg
							Glutamic acid	194 mg
							Glycine	15 mg
							Proline	10 mg
							Serine	25 mg

Green	Proximates		Vitamins		Minerals		Amino Acids	
Lettuce, Red leaf	Water	95.64 g	Vitamin A	7492 IU	Calcium	33 mg	Histidine	19 mg
	Protein	1.33 g	Vitamin B6	0.100 mg	Iron	1.20 mg	Isoleucine	38 mg
	Calories	16	Vitamin C	3.7 mg	Magnesium	12 mg	Leucine	70 mg
			Vitamin E	0.15 mg	Phosphorus	28 mg	Lysine	45 mg
			Vitamin K	140.3 µg	Potassium	187 mg	Methionine	16 mg
			Thiamin	0.064 mg	Sodium	25 mg	Phenylalaline	67 mg
			Riboflavin	0.077 mg	Zinc	0.20 mg	Threonine	48 mg
			Niacin	0.321 mg	Copper	0.028 mg	Tryptophan	22 mg
			Vitamin B5	0.144 mg	Manganese	0.203 mg	Valine	48 mg
			Folate	36 µg	Selenium	1.5 µg		

Green	Proximates		Vitamins		Minerals		Amino Acids	
Lettuce, Romaine	Water	94.61 g	Vitamin A	5807 IU	Calcium	33 mg	Histidine	21 mg
	Protein	1.23 g	Vitamin B6	0.074 mg	Iron	0.97 mg	Isoleucine	45 mg
	Calories	17	Vitamin C	24.0 mg	Magnesium	14 mg	Leucine	76 mg
			Vitamin E	0.13 mg	Phosphorus	30 mg	Lysine	64 mg
			Vitamin K	102.5 µg	Potassium	247 mg	Methionine	15 mg
			Thiamin	0.072 mg	Sodium	8 mg	Phenylalaline	65 mg
			Riboflavin	0.067 mg	Zinc	0.23 mg	Threonine	43 mg
			Niacin	0.313 mg	Copper	0.048 mg	Tryptophan	10 mg
			Vitamin B5	0.142 mg	Manganese	0.155 mg	Valine	55 mg
			Folate	136 µg	Selenium	0.4 µg		
Mint	Water	78.65 g	Vitamin A	4248 IU	Calcium	243 mg	Histidine	75 mg
	Protein	3.75 g	Vitamin B6	0.129 mg	Iron	5.08 mg	Isoleucine	154 mg
	Calories	44	Vitamin C	31.8 mg	Magnesium	80 mg	Leucine	281 mg
			Vitamin E	n/a	Phosphorus	73 mg	Lysine	161 mg
			Vitamin K	n/a	Potassium	569 mg	Methionine	53 mg
			Thiamin	0.082 mg	Sodium	31 mg	Phenylalaline	191 mg
			Riboflavin	0.266 mg	Zinc	1.11 mg	Threonine	154 mg
			Niacin	1.706 mg	Copper	0.329 mg	Tryptophan	58 mg
			Vitamin B5	0.338 mg	Manganese	1.176 mg	Valine	187 mg
			Folate	114 µg	Selenium	n/a		
Parsley	Water	87.71 g	Vitamin A	8424 IU	Calcium	138 mg	Histidine	61 mg
	Protein	2.97 g	Vitamin B6	0.090 mg	Iron	6.20 mg	Isoleucine	118 mg
	Calories	36	Vitamin C	133.0 mg	Magnesium	50 mg	Leucine	204 mg
			Vitamin E	0.75 mg	Phosphorus	58 mg	Lysine	181 mg
			Vitamin K	1640.0 µg	Potassium	554 mg	Methionine	42 mg
			Thiamin	0.086 mg	Sodium	56 mg	Phenylalaline	145 mg
			Riboflavin	0.098 mg	Zinc	1.07 mg	Threonine	122 mg
			Niacin	1.313 mg	Copper	0.149 mg	Tryptophan	45 mg
			Vitamin B5	0.400 mg	Manganese	0.160 mg	Valine	172 mg
			Folate	152 µg	Selenium	0.1 µg		
Spinach	Water	91.40 g	Vitamin A	9377 IU	Calcium	99 mg	Histidine	64 mg
	Protein	2.86 g	Vitamin B6	0.195 mg	Iron	2.71 mg	Isoleucine	147 mg
	Calories	23	Vitamin C	28.1 mg	Magnesium	79 mg	Leucine	223 mg
			Vitamin E	2.03 mg	Phosphorus	49 mg	Lysine	174 mg
			Vitamin K	482.9 µg	Potassium	558 mg	Methionine	53 mg
			Thiamin	0.078 mg	Sodium	79 mg	Phenylalaline	129 mg
			Riboflavin	0.189 mg	Zinc	0.53 mg	Threonine	122 mg
			Niacin	0.724 mg	Copper	0.130 mg	Tryptophan	39 mg
			Vitamin B5	0.065 mg	Manganese	0.897 mg	Valine	161 mg
			Folate	194 µg	Selenium	1.0 µg		
Watercress	Water	95.11 g	Vitamin C	43 mg	Calcium	120 mg	Tryptophan	30 mg
	Protein	2.3 g	Thiamin	.090 mg	Iron .	20 mg	Threonine	133 mg
	Calories	11	Riboflavin	.120 mg	Magnesium	21 mg	Isoleucine	93 mg
			Niacin	.200 mg	Phosphorus	60 mg	Leucine	166 mg
			Vitamin B6	.129 mg	Potassium	330 mg	Lysine	134 mg

Green	Proximates	Vitamins		Minerals		Amino Acids	
Watercress		Folate	9 µg	Sodium	41 mg	Methionine	20 mg
cont'd.		Vitamin A	31911 U	Zinc	.11 mg	Cystine	7 mg
		Vitamin E	1.00 mg			Phenylalanine	114 mg
		Vitamin K	250 µg			Tyrosine	63 mg
						Valine	137 mg
						Arginine	150 mg
						Histidine	40 mg
						Alanine	137 mg
						Glycine	112 mg
						Proline	96 mg
						Serine	60 mg

U.S. Department of Agriculture, Agricultural Research Service. 2007. USDA Nutrient Database for Standard Reference, Release 20. Nutrient Data Laboratory Home Page: http://www.ars.usda.gov/nutrientdata

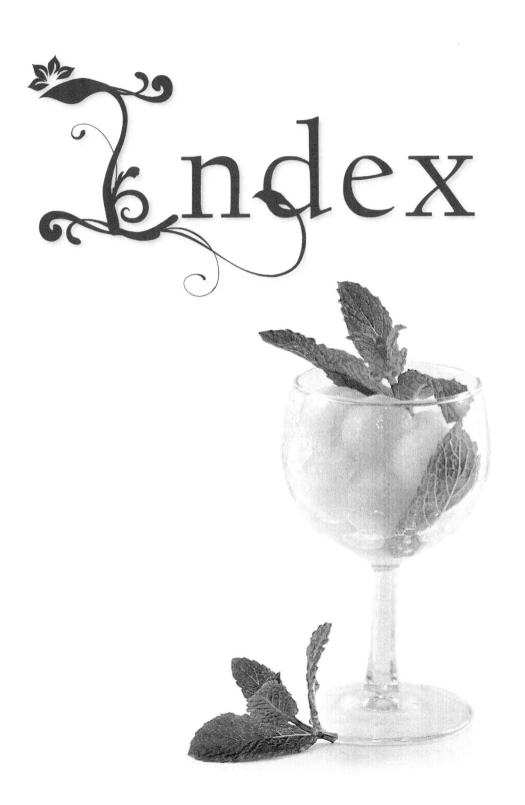

Index

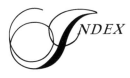 *INDEX*

29020799R00163

Made in the USA
Lexington, KY
11 January 2014